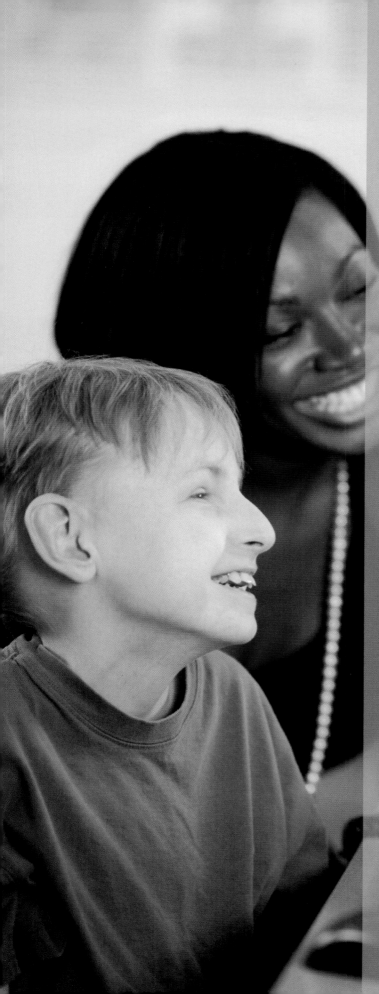

Learning Disability Nursing
at a Glance

Edited by

Bob Gates
Professor of Learning Disabilities
Institute for Practice, Interdisciplinary Research and Enterprise (INSPIRE)
University of West London; and
Emeritus Professor
The Centre for Learning Disability Studies
University of Hertfordshire; and Honorary
Professor of Learning Disabilities at the
Hertfordshire Partnership University NHS
Foundation Trust

Debra Fearns
Senior Lecturer and Field Lead for LD Nursing
Degree
The Centre for Learning Disability Studies
University of Hertfordshire

Jo Welch
Senior Lecturer
The Centre for Learning Disability Studies
University of Hertfordshire

WILEY Blackwell

Library of Congress Cataloging-in-Publication Data

Learning disability nursing at a glance / [edited by] Bob Gates, Debra Fearns, Jo Welch.
　　p. ; cm. – (At a glance series)
　　Includes bibliographical references and index.
　　ISBN 978-1-118-50613-4 (pbk.)
I. Gates, Bob, 1955- editor.　II. Fearns, Debra, editor.　III. Welch, Jo, editor.
IV. Series: At a glance series (Oxford, England)
　　[DNLM: 1. Learning Disorders–nursing. WY 160.5]
　　RC394.L37
　　616.85′8890231–dc23

2014023098

A catalogue record for this book is available from the British Library.

Wiley also publishes its books in a variety of electronic formats. Some content that appears in print may not be available in electronic books.

Cover image: © Christopher Futcher/i-Stock

Cover design by Meaden Creative

Set in 9.5/11.5pt Minion by SPi Publisher Services, Pondicherry, India
Printed and bound in Singapore by Markono Print Media Pte Ltd

1　2015

Contents

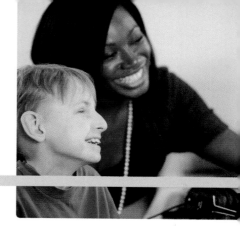

Contributors viii
Preface xi
How to use your revision guide xiii
About the companion website xvii

Part 1   Introduction to learning disability nursing   1

1   What is learning disability nursing?   2
2   Nursing and midwifery standards   4
3   The six Cs   6
4   The student nurse perspective   7

Part 2   Exploration of learning disability   9

5   What is a learning disability?   10
6   Causes of learning disability   12
7   Chromosomal disorders   14
8   Genetic disorders   16
9   Other causes of learning disability   18

Part 3   Childhood development   21

10   Screening and genetics   22
11   Developmental milestones   24
12   Common childhood diseases   26
13   Developing communication   28
14   Learning through play   30
15   Education   32
16   Screening for autistic spectrum conditions   34
17   Safeguarding children   36

Part 4   Adolescence   39

18   Puberty   40
19   Bullying   42
20   Child and adolescent mental health services   44
21   Transitions   46

Part 5   Adults with a learning disability   49

22   Working with adults with learning disability   50
23   Communicating with people with learning disability   52
24   Sensory impairment   54
25   Living with Autistic Spectrum Conditions   56
26   Epilepsy in adults with learning disability   58
27   Management of epilepsy   60

Part 6

People with a learning disability and additional mental health needs 63

28 Managing challenging behaviour 64
29 Mental health issues 66
30 Personality disorder 68
31 Offenders with a learning disability 70

Part 7

Vulnerable adults with a learning disability 73

32 Mental Capacity Act 74
33 Human rights 76
34 Equality Act 2010 78
35 Mental Health Act 80
36 Ethics, rights and responsibilities 82

Part 8

Biophysical aspects of learning disability nursing 85

37 Biophysical aspects of learning disabilities 86
38 Common health issues 88
39 The Health Action Plan 90
40 Pain assessment and recognition 92
41 Palliative and end-of-life care 94
42 Dementia in people with Down's syndrome 96
43 Sexual health issues 98
44 Postural care 100

Part 9

Older people with a learning disability 103

45 Older people with a learning disability 104
46 Dementia care 106
47 The Mental State Examination 108

Part 10

Medication 111

48 Antidepressant and antipsychotic drugs 112
49 Antiepileptic drugs 114
50 Nurse prescribing 116
51 Drug calculations 118

Part 11

The learning disability nurse 121

52 The community learning disability nurse 122
53 Healthcare facilitators 124
54 The health liaison nurse 126
55 The assessment and treatment learning disability nurse 128
56 The prison nurse 130

Part 12

Inclusion 133

57 Person centred planning 134
58 Employment 136
59 Housing and leisure 138
60 Ethnic minorities and learning disability 140
61 Parents with a learning disability 142

62 Family perspectives 144
63 A service user's perspective 146
64 Advocacy 148
65 Health passports 150
66 Hate crime 151
67 Sex and individuals with a learning disability 152
68 Spirituality 154
69 The twenty-first century: Networking for success 155

Further reading and resources 157
Index 161

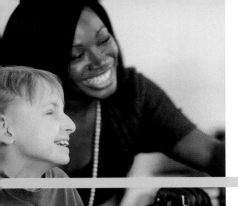

Contributors

Samuel Abdulla
Community Learning Disability Nurse
Associate Lecturer in Learning Disability Nursing
Edinburgh Napier University

Vicky Avellino
RNLD
Senior Nurse Team leader
Southern Health Foundation NHS Trust

Carol Bailey
Consultant Nurse: Learning Disabilities
Clinical Service Director (Hampshire)
Learning Disability Division
Southern Health NHS Foundation Trust

Jo Ball
Senior Occupational Therapist
Solent NHS Trust

Cheryl Beatie
Honorary Fellow
School of Nursing (Learning Disability)
University of Hertfordshire

Deborah Birtchnell
Nursing Sister
HMP The Mount
Hertfordshire

Diana Boyce
Senior Locality Community Learning Disability Nurse
Southern Health NHS Foundation Trust

Jenna Braddick
Speech and Language Therapist
Hertfordshire Partnership Foundation Trust

Noel Burke
Community Learning Disabilities Staff Nurse
Southampton City Community Learning Disability Team

Claudia Camden-Smith
Higher Specialty Trainee in Psychiatry of Intellectual
Disability
Wessex Deanery

Emily Casserly
Nurse Practitioner, RNMH
Edinburgh Napier University

Rebecca Chester
Professional Lead Nurse – Learning Disabilities
Berkshire Healthcare NHS Foundation Trust
Lecturer Practitioner in Learning Disability Nursing
the Centre for Learning Disability Studies
University of Hertfordshire

Anita Claridge-Lawrence
Sexual Health Facilitator (Learning Disability)
North Essex

David Clark
Student Learning Disability Nurse
University of Hertfordshire

Sarah Clayton
Managing Director
Postural Care Community Interest Company

Christine Cole
Clinical Epilepsy Specialist Nurse
Barnet Learning Disability Service
Central London Community Health Care

Natasha Collins
Community Learning Disability Nurse
Adult Learning Disability Team
Bedford Borough Council

Ruth Cooper
Clinical Nurse Specialist – Sensory Impairment, and
Independent Nurse Prescriber
Services for People who have a Learning Disability
South Essex Partnership NHS Foundation Trust

Lisa Dexter
Community Learning Disability Nurse Specialist (North Essex)
Hertfordshire Partnership University Foundation Trust

Jennifer Dolman
Consultant Psychiatrist Learning Disabilities
Southern Health NHS Foundation Trust

Mary Donnelly
Senior Lecturer in Children's Health
University of Hertfordshire

Terri Dorman
Clinical Group Manager for Learning Disability
Services for People who have a Learning Disability (SEPT)
Bedfordshire

Catherine Dunne
Student Health Visitor
the Centre for Learning Disability Studies
University of Hertfordshire

Debra Fearns
Senior Lecturer
Learning Disability Nursing
the Centre for Learning Disability Studies
University of Hertfordshire

Joanne Fisher-Joannides
Forensic Liaison Nurse
Hertfordshire Partnership NHS Foundation Trust
HMP The Mount

Natasha Fletcher
Community Nurse (Learning Disability)
Adult Learning Disability Team (ALDT)
Bedford Borough Council

Sarah Futcher
Community Learning Disabilities Staff Nurse
Southampton

Bob Gates
Professor of Learning Disabilities
Institute for Practice, Interdisciplinary Research
and Enterprise (INSPIRE)
University of West London; and
Emeritus Professor
The Centre for Learning Disability Studies
University of Hertfordshire

Elizabeth Gormley-Fleming
Principal Lecturer, Learning and Teaching
Senior Lecturer, Children's Nursing
University of Hertfordshire

Aidan Graham
Senior Nurse Practitioner, RNLD
Bluebird House
Bournemouth University

James Hawkins
Deputy CEO
Young People's Service Manager
Respond
London

Sarah Holmes
Community Learning Disability Nurse
Bedford Borough Council

Joanne James
Company Director of EC Consultancy Ltd
Rotherham School of Nursing
University of Sheffield

Jennifer Jones
Southampton City Community Learning Disability Team

Nichola Keer
Adult Safeguarding Lead Nurse
Bedford Hospital

Sandra Kelly
Lead Community Learning Disability Nurse (North)
Cambridge and Peterborough Foundation
Trust (CPFT)

Amanda Keighley
Principal Lecturer/Academic Group Lead
the Centre for Learning Disability Studies
University of Hertfordshire

Paul Maloret
Senior Lecturer in Learning Disabilities
University of Hertfordshire

Daniel Marsden
Practice Development Nurse for People with
Learning Disabilities
East Kent Hospitals University NHS
Foundation Trust
William Harvey Hospital
Ashford

Gweneth Moulster
Clinical Director/Consultant Nurse
South Staffordshire and Shropshire NHS
Foundation Trust;
Honorary Teaching Fellow
University of Hertfordshire

Helen Murray
Visiting Lecturer
University of Hertfordshire

David O'Driscoll
Psychotherapist
Specialist Learning Disability Service
Hertfordshire Partnership University
NHS Foundation Trust;
Visiting Research Fellow
the Centre for Learning Disability Studies
University of Hertfordshire

Mary O'Toole
Sibling to Anne, who has Learning Disabilities
Honorary Fellow (Family Advocate)
the Centre for Learning Disability Studies
University of Hertfordshire

Michelle Parker
RNLD Exemplar Health Care
University of York

Maggie Jones
Senior Lecturer in Learning Disability Nursing
the Centre for Learning Disability Studies
University of Hertfordshire

Sheila Roberts
Senior Lecturer in Children's Nursing
University of Hertfordshire

Florence Sayekaya
Forensic Specialist Nurse Practitioner, Learning Disabilities
Southern Health NHS Trust

Tracey-Jo Simpson
Visiting Lecturer
the Centre for Learning Disability Studies
University of Hertfordshire

Paul Smith
Transition Nurse
Royal Free NHS Foundation Trust.
Visiting Lecturer in Learning Disability Nursing
the Centre for Learning Disability Studies
University of Hertfordshire

Rooja Sooben
Visiting Lecturer in Learning Disability
University of Hertfordshire

Mohammad Surfraz
Senior Lecturer
Learning Disability Nursing
School of Health and Social Work
the Centre for Learning Disability Studies
University of Hertfordshire

Gamuchirayi Tendayi
Senior Lecturer in Learning Disability Nursing
the Centre for Learning Disability Studies
University of Hertfordshire

Melanie Webb
Locality Senior Nurse North Hampshire / Nurse Prescriber
Learning Disability Division
Southern Health Foundation NHS Trust

Anne Webster
Manager/ Learning Disability nurse, Hertfordshire Partnership
University NHS Foundation Trust.
Honorary Fellow
the Centre for Learning Disability Studies
University of Hertfordshire

David Weinrabe
Formerly Principal Lecturer in Learning Disability
Nursing and Healthcare
University of Hertfordshire

Jo Welch
Senior Lecturer Learning Disability Nursing
Facilitator Positive Choices Network
the Centre for Learning Disability Studies
University of Hertfordshire

Alison Williamson
Senior Lecturer in Learning Disability Nursing
the Centre for Learning Disability Studies
University of Hertfordshire

Sally Wilson
Acute Liaison Nurse
Coventry and Warwickshire Partnership Trust

Melissa Wilton
Staff Nurse
Hertfordshire Partnership University NHS
Foundation Trust

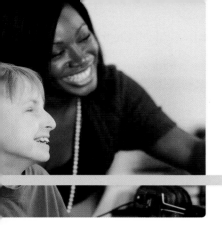

Preface

It is with enormous pride that we offer this new and exciting book – *Learning Disability Nursing at a Glance*; one that is in a series of popular nursing texts. The aim of this book is to provide learning disability nursing students with user-friendly, contemporary information in relation to some of the key clinical practice issues that they may encounter when working with people with learning disabilities. At the outset we need to make clear our use of terminology in this text. Generally speaking within the UK, the term *'learning disability'* is used to describe people with significant developmental delay that results in arrested or incomplete achievement of the *'normal'* milestones of human development. The term 'learning disabilities' is also used elsewhere throughout the world, but it holds different meanings in many other countries; paradoxically so too in the UK. It is this difference in meaning that causes confusion to, what we hope, will be an international audience of readers. Elsewhere in the world alternative terms to *'learning disability'* are used, such as 'mental retardation', and 'mental handicap', but these terms are felt to portray negative imagery concerning people with learning disabilities. There are more positive international terms in use, such as 'intellectual disability' and 'developmental disability' but we have decided to adopt the consistent use of a term which we believe seems most appropriate to this text, and for the readership, as well as those who this book is principally about, and that is *'learning disability'*. Therefore, throughout the remainder of this book we will only use the term learning disability, save where certain Acts and, or, other technical works require other terminology for accuracy.

The text has been edited using expert contributions from learning disability academic staff as well as clinicians. While there are currently a number of texts available that describe nursing practice from an adult perspective, there are few that deal with practice specifically related to people with learning disabilities. And indeed fewer still that address the needs of people with learning disabilities across the life spectrum, from children through to adolescents and on to adults and older people. Also, many of the current texts related to people with learning disabilities that are available tend to deal with the subject of *learning disabilities*, rather than *learning disability nursing*; this book does both. Uniquely, the book is aimed at health and social care students, as well as registered nurses, but will be of use to a wide range of other students from a wide variety of vocational, academic and professional backgrounds, and other fields of nursing. Principally the book is intended to provide nursing students with material that is accessible, up to date, and readily available. The text addresses the principles underpinning contemporary learning disability nursing practice that students are likely to encounter, and these are discussed in the context of maintaining health and wellbeing. And in order to reflect the contemporary field of learning disability nursing practice, the text embraces both primary and secondary care perspectives. Learning disability nurses can now be found working and supporting people in diverse care contexts, such as community learning disability teams, treatment and assessment services, outreach services, residential settings, day care and respite services, health facilitation and hospital liaison roles, mental health and, or, challenging behaviour services, special schools and specialist services for people who can be located on the spectrum of autistic conditions. Additionally, they can be found working for many different agencies and organisations, such as health, social care, education and the independent sector (this comprises the private, voluntary and not-for-profit organisations), and also alongside numerous other professional disciplines that include clinical psychologists, social workers, occupational therapists, speech and language therapists, and consultant psychiatrists in learning disabilities as well as a range of professionals within mainstream health, social services and education. Given this complexity, there is need for a text that holds an overarching aim of helping learning disability nursing students understand fundamental aspects of their practice, in order to provide safe, effective and compassionate care to people with learning disabilities in a variety of situations. From an academic perspective, there is often a lot of support available to learning disability nursing students for their academic assessment and progression. However, when in practice, learning disability nursing students may find themselves being supervised from a distance and, as such, this proposed text could accompany them in a variety of settings to assist their integration of theory and practice. This text is based upon the principles of care; a foundation text to encourage the learning disability nursing student to grow and develop.

The book has been designed to be used as a quick reference guide in either practice settings, educational establishments or at home and has been written in easy-to-understand language, drawing heavily on diagrams and pictures to support visual learners. Therefore it is not intended that you read this book from cover to cover in one sitting, rather – as its name implies – the text should be seen as an 'at a glance' guide or manual.

The book is divided into 12 parts, each containing a variable number of chapters that relate to the theme of that part. The parts of the book include: an introduction to learning disability nursing, an exploration of learning disability, childhood development, adolescence, adults with a learning disability, people with a learning disability and additional mental health needs, vulnerable adults with a learning disability, biophysical aspects of learning disability nursing, older people with a learning disability, medication, the learning disability nurse and issues of inclusion.

We hope that *Learning Disability Nursing At A Glance* will come to be seen as a highly regarded textbook, not only in the field of learning disabilities but also more widely, and that it will be used widely by the many professionals and students from a wide range of different professional and academic backgrounds. We believe that the excellent end product that you have before you is due, in no small part, to the excellent contributions that have been made by our many friends and colleagues across the UK and Southern Ireland, and we offer our thanks for contributing to this book. We hope that you find the book helpful and that through using it, in some small way, it assists you in supporting people with learning disabilities enjoy good health and wellbeing in their lives.

Bob Gates
Debra Fearns
Jo Welch

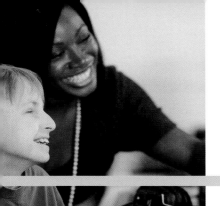

How to use your revision guide

Features contained within your revision guide

The overview page gives a summary of the topics covered in each part.

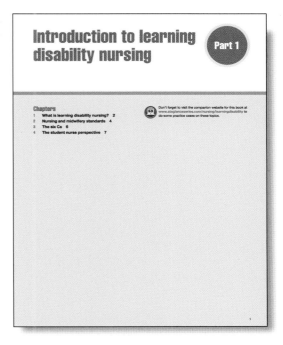

Each topic is presented in a double-page spread with clear, easy-to-follow diagrams supported by succinct explanatory text.

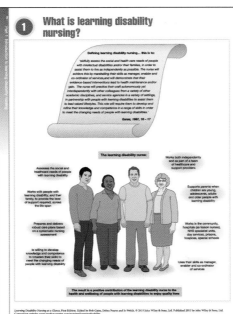

Summary boxes remind you about key points to remember.

Summary

- Chromosomes are made of DNA.
- Each contains genes in a linear order.
- Human body cells contain 46 chromosomes in 23 pairs – one of each pair inherited from each parent.
- Chromosome pairs 1–22 are called autosomes.
- The 23rd pair are called sex chromosomes: XX is female, XY is male.

The website icon indicates that you can find accompanying resources on the book's companion website.

The anytime, anywhere textbook

Wiley E-Text

Your book is also available to purchase as a **Wiley E-Text: Powered by VitalSource** version – a digital, interactive version of this book which you own as soon as you download it.

Your **Wiley E-Text** allows you to:

Search: Save time by finding terms and topics instantly in your book, your notes, even your whole library (once you've downloaded more textbooks)

Note and Highlight: Colour code, highlight and make digital notes right in the text so you can find them quickly and easily

Organize: Keep books, notes and class materials organized in folders inside the application

Share: Exchange notes and highlights with friends, classmates and study groups

Upgrade: Your textbook can be transferred when you need to change or upgrade computers

Link: Link directly from the page of your interactive textbook to all of the material contained on the companion website

The **Wiley E-Text** version will also allow you to copy and paste any photograph or illustration into assignments, presentations and your own notes.

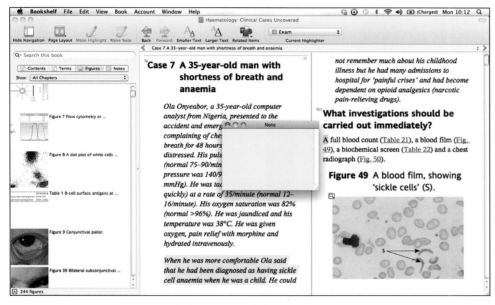

Wiley E-Text
Powered by VitalSource®

To access your Wiley E-Text:

- Visit **www.vitalsource.com/software/bookshelf/downloads** to download the Bookshelf application to your computer, laptop, tablet or mobile device.
- Open the Bookshelf application on your computer and register for an account.
- Follow the registration process.

CourseSmart

CourseSmart gives you instant access (via computer or mobile device) to this Wiley-Blackwell e-book and its extra electronic functionality, at 40% off the recommended retail print price. See all the benefits at: **www.coursesmart.com/students**

Instructors … receive your own digital desk copies!

CourseSmart also offers instructors an immediate, efficient, and environmentally-friendly way to review this book for your course.

For more information visit **www.coursesmart.com/instructors**.

With CourseSmart, you can create lecture notes quickly with copy and paste, and share pages and notes with your students. Access your **CourseSmart** digital book from your computer or mobile device instantly for evaluation, class preparation, and as a teaching tool in the classroom.

Simply sign in at **http://instructors.coursesmart.com/bookshelf** to download your Bookshelf and get started. To request your desk copy, hit 'Request Online Copy' on your search results or book product page.

We hope you enjoy using your new book. Good luck with your studies!

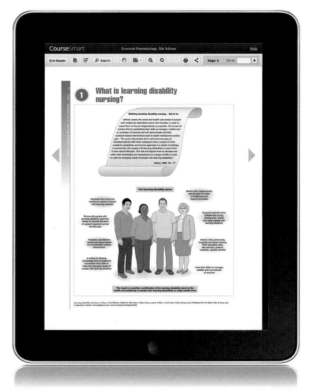

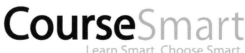

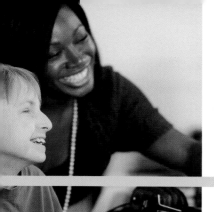

About the companion website

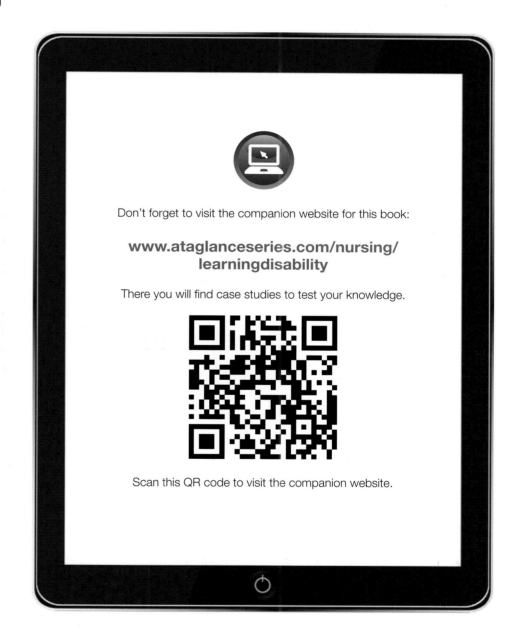

Don't forget to visit the companion website for this book:

**www.ataglanceseries.com/nursing/
learningdisability**

There you will find case studies to test your knowledge.

Scan this QR code to visit the companion website.

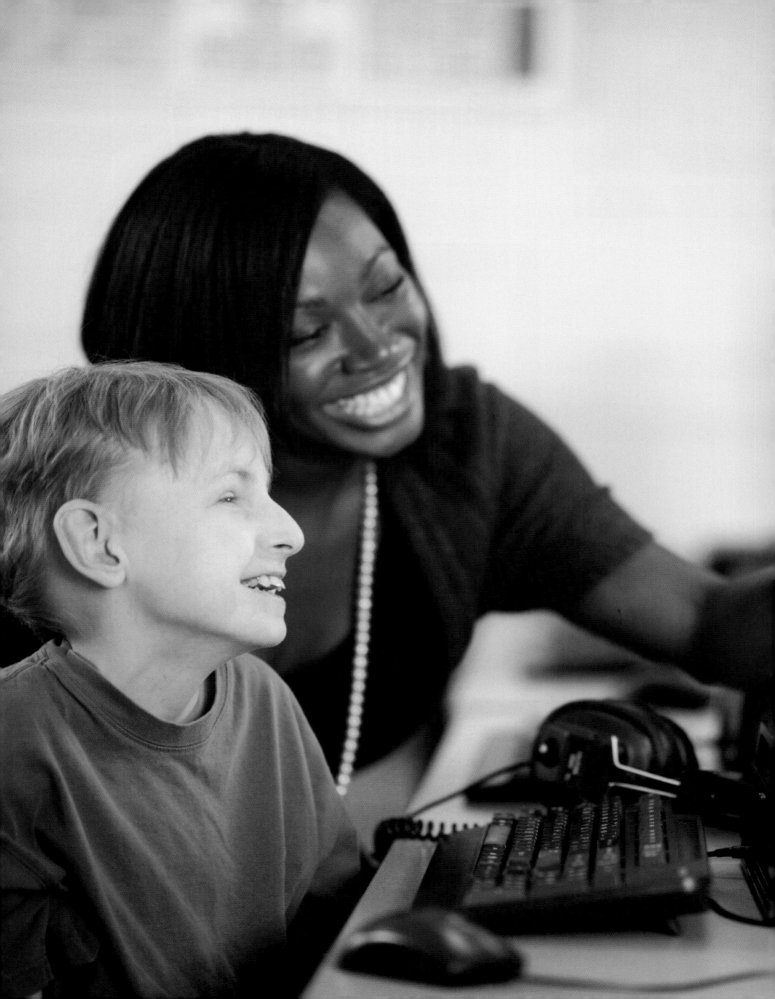

Introduction to learning disability nursing

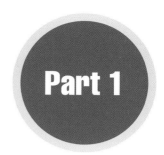

Part 1

Chapters

1   **What is learning disability nursing?**   2
2   **Nursing and midwifery standards**   4
3   **The six Cs**   6
4   **The student nurse perspective**   7

Don't forget to visit the companion website for this book at
www.ataglanceseries.com/nursing/learningdisability to
do some practice cases on these topics.

1 What is learning disability nursing?

Defining learning disability nursing… this is to:

'skilfully assess the social and health care needs of people with learning disabilities and, or, this families, in order to assist them to live as independently as possible. The nurse will achieve this by marshalling their skills as manager, enabler and co-ordinator of services, and will demonstrate that their evidence-based interventions lead to health maintenance and/or gain. The nurse will practice their craft autonomously yet interdependently with other colleagues from a variety of other academic disciplines, and service agencies in a variety of settings, in partnership with people with learning disabilities to assist them to lead valued lifestyles. This role will require them to develop and refine their knowledge and competence in a range of skills in order to meet the changing needs of people with learning disabilities.'

Gates, 1997, 16 – 17

The learning disability nurse:

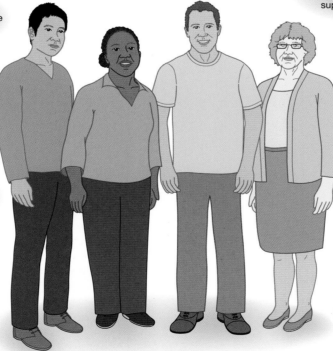

Assesses the social and healthcare needs of people with learning disability

Works with people with learning disability, and their family, to provide the level of support required, across the life span

Prepares and delivers robust care plans based on a systematic nursing assessment

Is willing to develop knowledge and competence to broaden their skills to meet the changing needs of people with learning disability

Works both independently and as part of a team of healthcare and support providers

Supports parents when children are young, adolescents, adults and older people with learning disability

Works in the community, hospitals (as liaison nurses), NHS specialist units, day services, prisons, hospices, special schools

Uses their skills as manager, enabler and co-ordinator of services

The result is a positive contribution of the learning disability nurse to the health and wellbeing of people with learning disabilities to enjoy quality lives

Learning Disability Nursing at a Glance, First Edition. Edited by Bob Gates, Debra Fearns and Jo Welch. © 2015 John Wiley & Sons, Ltd. Published 2015 by John Wiley & Sons, Ltd.
Companion website: www.ataglanceseries.com/nursing/learningdisability

Introduction

Learning disability nursing is a person-centred profession whose primary aim is to support people with learning disabilities either directly or indirectly through improving or maintaining their health and wellbeing, and bringing about their social inclusion in their communities.

What do learning disability nurses do?

Learning disability nurses work with people with learning disabilities from birth through to death, those who may require a range of supports throughout their lives. This support will range from none, or minimal, support through to intensive holistic nursing care aimed at meeting the multidimensional needs of people with learning disabilities. Much of the care planning and delivery of learning disability takes place in local community settings. Learning disability nurses must be competent in preparing robust, professionally prepared care plans based on a systematic nursing assessment. Much evidence exists of the positive contribution of learning disability nurses to the lives of people with learning disabilities. Learning disability nurses currently work in a wide range of organisational settings that include the NHS, local authorities and the third sector. Typically they are likely to work in inter-professional teams and for a variety of agencies. Recent changes in health and social care are dictating new and exciting roles that are being undertaken by learning disability nurses, for example nurses working in mainstream healthcare teams in acute hospitals, mental health services and primary care. The *Strengthening the Commitment Learning Disability Nursing* (UK, Chief Nursing Officers, 2012) report has asserted that learning disability nurses are needed to ensure that people with learning disabilities of all ages, today and tomorrow, have access to the expert learning disabilities nursing they need, want and deserve. Three primary areas of practice in the NHS are:

- Health facilitation – supporting mainstream access.
- Inpatient services – for example, assessment and treatment, and secure services.
- Specialist roles – in community learning disability teams.

Other, broader, developments in healthcare roles, such as the modern matron, specialist epilepsy nurses and nurse prescribers are all providing new areas of practice for learning disability nurses. Also learning disability nurses work as consultants who are able to offer valuable clinical, supervisory expertise along with both regional and national professional leadership.

The purist form of nursing – the context of learning disability nursing

Learning disability nursing is often referred to as the purist form of nursing; unlike colleagues in other fields of nursing, they do not concentrate on specific manifestations of physical ill health or trauma, or mental health and wellbeing, or children, or childbirth for that matter; rather they offer support to people with learning disabilities, and their families that is all embracing and quite literally from the cradle through to the grave. In order to offer competent, compassionate and comprehensive nursing interventions that meet the multidimensional needs of people with learning disability, it is helpful to adopt a structured approach to working. A comprehensive needs assessment (physical, psychological, social, spiritual and emotional) should first be completed. If a nurse is required to work with someone with learning disabilities and their family, it is necessary that their needs are assessed and incorporated into an individual care plan, taking their desires, wishes and aspirations into account. The nurse must work closely with the client's family, care providers, and other professionals, as this approach will bring very important and essential information, as well as informing the development of a care plan, its approach, delivery and management. This detailed assessment is followed by the construction of a written care plan that is implemented, and followed up with ongoing review/s and evaluation/s. This very structured approach, using partnership working, and incorporating the multidimensionality of people, coupled with the person at the heart of planning, ensures that learning disability nurses provide holistic person-centred care and support.

A modelled approach

In response to social and political influences, learning disability care and models of support, care planning has changed considerably over recent years, as has the practice of learning disability nurses. For example, during the last century, many people with learning disabilities were located in asylums and, or, long-stay hospitals that were dominated by a medical model of care, emphasising the biological needs of people, and the need to 'cure' physical problems. Most people with learning disabilities have now moved out of long-stay hospitals, but there remains a concern that the powerful effects of the medical model may continue to influence care provided in smaller community-based residences. It has been argued that the use of the medical model in the past pathologised and objectified people with learning disabilities, leading to them being seen as 'less than human'. Therefore, nurses need to consider adopting a 'nursing model' to guide their care in practice, to ensure that they offer holistic nursing support. The use of any model must hold the person with learning disabilities central to the care planning process, and all must be mindful that they use a model to promote what is best for that person. There are numerous nursing models that can be adapted and used in health and social care settings. Some nursing models are regularly used in learning disability nursing practice. An example of a useful nursing model is that of Roper, Logan and Tierney (2002) this is well known and widely used within nursing profession. The model focuses on holistic care and is based on the concept of health rather than illness and disease. The model focuses on understanding the needs of people in terms of the activities of daily living they perform. The model embraces the idea that independence and dependence operate along a continuum relating to each activity of living separately.

Nursing and midwifery standards

Nursing and Midwifery Council standards for pre-registration nursing: learning disability nursing

All nurses and midwives are required to comply with The Code: Standards of conduct, performance and ethics for nurses and midwives (NMC 2008) (the code)

The public can be confident that all new nurses will deliver high quality essential care to all deliver complex care to service users in their field of practice

Act to safeguard the public, and be responsible and accountable for safe, person-centred, evidence-based nursing practice

Act with professionalism and integrity, and work within agreed professional, ethical and legal frameworks and processes to maintain and improve standards

Practise in a compassionate, respectful way, maintaining dignity and wellbeing and communicating effectively

Act on their understanding of how people's lifestyles, environments and the location of care delivery influence their health and wellbeing

Seek out every opportunity to promote health and prevent illness

Work in partnership with other health and social care professionals and agencies, service users, carers and families ensuring that decisions about care are shared

Use leadership skills to supervise and manage others and contribute to planning, designing, delivering and improving future services

Nurses must be able to meet all NMC requirements when they qualify and then maintain their knowledge and skills

The following outlines specific learning disability competencies for entry onto the NMC register and is not a comprehensive guide to ALL the nursing requirements necessary for registration (2010).

Learning disability nursing: specific competencies for entry to the register

Professional values

Learning disabilities nurses must promote the individuality, independence, rights, choice and social inclusion of people with learning disabilities and highlight their strengths and abilities at all times while encouraging others do the same. They must facilitate the active participation of families and carers.

Learning disabilities nurses must understand and apply current legislation to all service users, paying special attention to the protection of vulnerable people, including those with complex needs arising from ageing, cognitive impairment, long-term conditions and those approaching the end of life.

Learning disabilities nurses must always promote the autonomy, rights and choices of people with learning disabilities and support and involve their families and carers, ensuring that each person's rights are upheld according to policy and the law.

Learning disabilities nurses must use their knowledge and skills to exercise professional advocacy, and recognise when it is appropriate to refer to independent advocacy services to safeguard dignity and human rights.

Learning disabilities nurses must recognise that people with learning disabilities are full and equal citizens, and must promote their health and wellbeing by focusing on and developing their strengths and abilities.

Communication and interpersonal skills

Learning disabilities nurses must use complex communication and interpersonal skills and strategies to work with people of all ages who have learning disabilities and help them to express themselves. They must also be able to communicate and negotiate effectively with other professionals, services and agencies, and ensure that people with learning disabilities, their families and carers, are fully involved in decision-making.

Learning disabilities nurses must use the full range of person-centred alternative and augmentative communication strategies and skills to build partnerships and therapeutic relationships with people with learning disabilities.

Learning disabilities nurses must be able to make all relevant information accessible to and understandable by people with learning disabilities, including adaptation of format, presentation and delivery.

Learning disabilities nurses must use a structured approach to assess, communicate with, interpret and respond therapeutically to people with learning disabilities who have complex physical and psychological health needs or those in behavioural distress.

Learning disabilities nurses must recognise and respond therapeutically to the complex behaviour that people with learning disabilities may use as a means of communication.

Nursing practice and decision making

• *Learning disabilities nurses* must have an enhanced knowledge of the health and developmental needs of all people with learning disabilities, and the factors that might influence them.

They must aim to improve and maintain their health and independence through skilled direct and indirect nursing care. They must also be able to provide direct care to meet the essential and complex physical and mental health needs of people with learning disabilities.

• *Learning disabilities nurses* must be able to recognise and respond to the needs of all people who come into their care including babies, children and young people, pregnant and postnatal women, people with mental health problems, people with physical health problems and disabilities, older people, and people with long-term problems such as cognitive impairment.

• *Learning disabilities nurses* must use a structured, person-centred approach to assess, interpret and respond therapeutically to people with learning disabilities, and their often complex, pre-existing physical and psychological health needs. They must work in partnership with service users, carers and other professionals, services and agencies to agree and implement individual care plans and ensure continuity of care.

• *Learning disabilities nurses* must lead the development, implementation and review of individual plans for all people with learning disabilities, to promote their optimum health and wellbeing and facilitate their equal access to all health, social care and specialist services.

• *Learning disabilities nurses* must work in partnership with people with learning disabilities and their families and carers to facilitate choice and maximise self-care and self-management and coordinate the transition between different services and agencies.

Leadership, management and team working

• *Learning disabilities nurses* must exercise collaborative management, delegation and supervision skills to create manage and support therapeutic environments for people with learning disabilities.

• *Learning disabilities nurses* must take the lead in ensuring that people with learning disabilities receive support that creatively addresses their physical, social, economic, psychological, spiritual and other needs, when assessing, planning and delivering care.

• *Learning disabilities nurses* must provide direction through leadership and education to ensure that their unique contribution is recognised in service design and provision.

• *Learning disabilities nurses* must use data and research findings on the health of people with learning disabilities to help improve people's experiences and care outcomes, and shape future services.

• *Learning disabilities nurses* must use leadership, influencing and decision-making skills to engage effectively with a range of agencies and professionals. They must also be able, when needed, to represent the health needs and protect the rights of people with learning disabilities and challenge negative stereotypes.

• *Learning disabilities nurses* must work closely with stakeholders to enable people with learning disabilities to exercise choice and challenge discrimination.

3 The six Cs

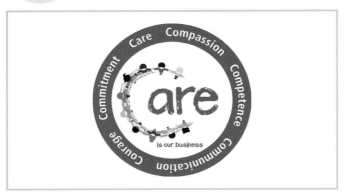

We need a common patient centered culture which produces, at the very least, the fundamental standards of care to which we are all entitled, at the same time as celebrating and supporting the provision of excellence in healthcare, (Francis, 2013).

Compassionate care and nursing makes all the difference to the experience of individuals. This requires that safe, high quality, compassionate care must be at the heart of everything we do, continually striving to improve, and speaking out if they witness standards which are wholly unacceptable.

Essential to creating a positive culture of safe, compassionate care is real, effective staff engagement to meet the demands of Francis. Compassionate care must be at the centre of everything the NHS does. This involves a clear and well-functioning system of accountability.

Safeguarding the health and wellbeing of those in your care means these people should not be exposed to abuse. Abuse is defined as 'a violation of an individual's human and civil rights by any other person or persons'. (No Secrets, DOH, 2000/Raising concerns: Guidance for nurses and midwives, NMC, 2013)

The 6 Cs

Care

Care is our core business and that of our organisation and the care we deliver helps the individual person and improves the health of the whole community. Caring defines us and our work. People receiving care expect it to be right for them, consistently, throughout every stage of their life.

Compassion

Compassion is how care is given through relationships based on empathy, respect and dignity – it can also be described as intelligent kindness, and is central to how people perceive their care.

Competence

Competence means all those in caring roles must have the ability to understand an individual's health and social needs and the expertise, clinical and technical knowledge to deliver effective care and treatments based on research and evidence.

Communication

Communication is central to successful caring relationships and to effective team working. Listening is as important as what we say and do and essential for 'no decision about me without me'. Communication is the key to a good workplace with benefits for those in our care and staff alike.

Courage

Courage enables us to do the right thing for the people we care for, to speak up when we have concerns and to have the personal strength and vision to innovate and to embrace new ways of working.

Commitment

A commitment to our patients and populations is a cornerstone of what we do. We need to build on our commitment to improve the care and experience of our patients, to take action to make this vision and strategy a reality for all and meet the health, care and support challenges ahead.

Why the 6Cs are needed

In order to maximise wellbeing and improve health outcomes, we will develop skills as health promoting practitioners, making every contact count for people. Learning disability nurses work in ways to reduce the health inequalities experienced by people with a learning disability and consider quality of care is as important as the quality of treatment. When a person reflects on their contact with a nurse they think about other issues as well – the environment they received care in; whether they were treated kindly, with respect and dignity; and whether they had to tell their story more than once. The people that we care for, and in many instances their families and carers, are our partners in care and our practice must reflect that. We must take note of:
- Person-centred Planning
- The Mental Capacity Act 2005
- Death by Indifference (2007)
- Health Care for All (2008)

People with learning disabilities are 58 times more likely to die before the age of 50 than the general population (Disability Rights Commission, 2006).

4 The student nurse perspective

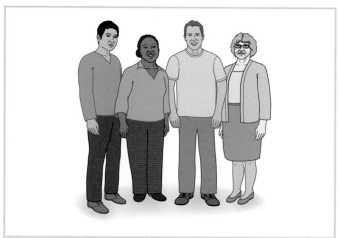

Universal issues

There are issues that are universal to all higher education undergraduate students, such as taking three years out of your life with no guarantees about what a degree may mean for the future. However, the education and learning processes prepare us to be lifelong learners – which everyone needs to be to advance career aspirations and goals. Then there are the challenges of negotiating your way around a large geographical area with seemingly endless corridors that feel like they go nowhere you need to be! And also developing the necessary skills to access the computer network; this is where you communicate with the university with regards to registration, modules, timetables and contacting tutors.

Student nurse issues

There are particular considerations in being a student nurse; unlike most students our fees are funded by the National Health Service and we are also paid a bursary. However, we work in real environments with real people. We study a longer academic year compared with non-nursing students: 47 weeks a year not 39. Doing assignments and reflective work can be difficult when you start but gets easier and improves our practice as time goes on and there is lots of advice available should you choose to access it.

Nursing is a value-based vocation. The Nursing and Midwifery Council (NMC) set out a statutory framework and publishes guidance from which we work. The NMC decide upon our training needs, they set out rules about our expected behaviours wherever we are in our professional and private lives. The Royal College of Nursing (RCN) represents all student and qualified nurses in respect of working conditions and pay. The RCN publishes guidelines about private and professional standards of behaviour. The RCN provides telephone and face-to-face personal representation. The RCN publishes journals for every imaginable type of nurse, from students in discrete fields to very senior managers; these publications provide access to further training and development.

Individual circumstances

There are also our individual circumstances: students in our groups range from recent school leavers to the more mature. Group members bring different qualities, experiences and motivations for wanting to be learning disabilities nurses. They represent many ethnic backgrounds, and have unique domestic circumstances; we have found that students develop supportive relationships, including study and revision groups.

The service user

Then there are the patients, clients and service users … labelled according to the placement setting. The fun and interesting part for us is getting to know all the people we are going to work with; and recognising that people who have learning disabilities invest time and energy in developing relationships with us too. This can represent the main privileges and responsibilities of the training. As students, we become aware that people who have learning disabilities may have had a long care career with frequent staff turnover which can impact their lives. We hope the frequent rotation of student nurses introduces positive and interesting experiences for them. We get to know peoples' most intimate information, become involved in their intimate care, their social and family networks; we get to write about their daily lives and relationships. This all requires skills, knowledge and values to respect the individuality and confidentiality of the person we are working with.

Placements

Going out to placement settings can be an exciting and challenging opportunity. We need to slot in, and to find our place, quickly in long established teams for relatively short periods of time. At the same time we are trying to reconcile and link theory and practice whilst getting skills 'signed off.' We have a lot of competencies to accomplish and we need to satisfy our mentors that we are safe practitioners. Mentors are continually assessing our progress from their own observations or those of the qualified staff that we work with. At the end of placement, mentors provide a professional written opinion on the skills, knowledge and values that we have demonstrated. This is a permanent record about our achievements. An important consideration of being on placement is that we are working with potential colleagues and employers, and as we come closer to qualifying this becomes more significant. Student nurses' education and training records have a significant purpose with an end view to us becoming competent and reliable practitioners. Due to this we feel that it is important to begin with, and continue to present, a professional approach to the academic and practical aspects of the training. Finally, we think that attending tutorials regularly and submitting assignments on time demonstrates time management and organisational skills. Also, being punctual in placement and attending every shift demonstrates the value of commitment; whilst using evidence-based practice ensures good quality service delivery, and this demonstrates knowledge.

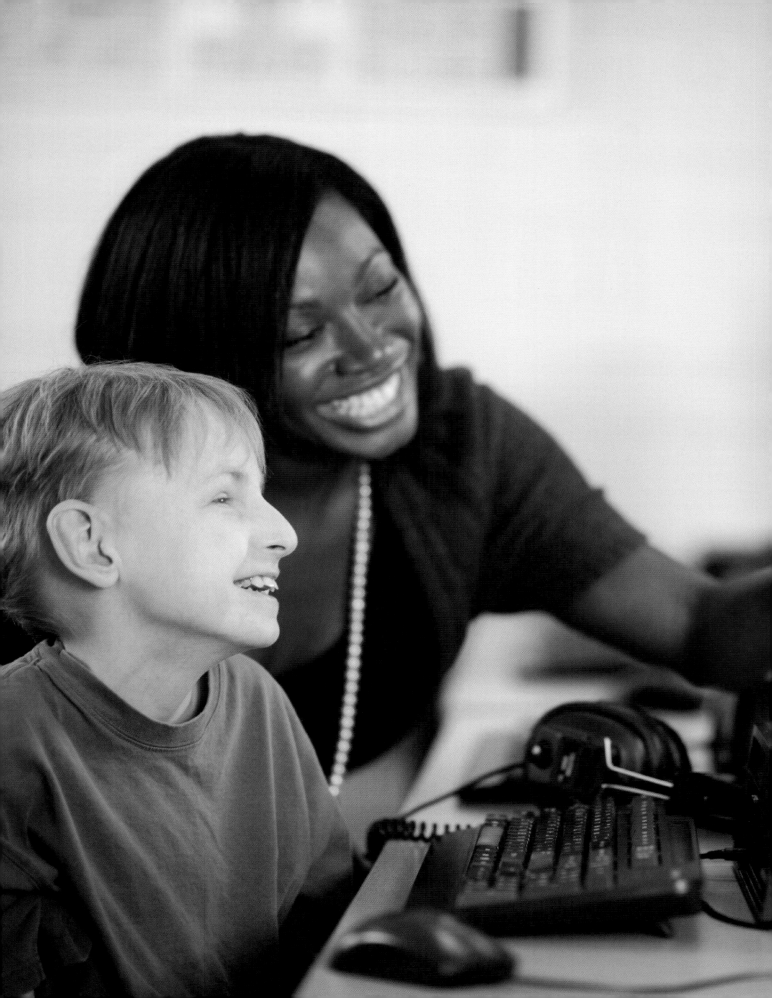

Exploration of learning disability

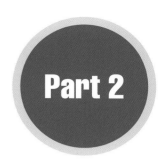

Part 2

Chapters

5   **What is a learning disability?**   10
6   **Causes of learning disability**   12
7   **Chromosomal disorders**   14
8   **Genetic disorders**   16
9   **Other causes of learning disability**   18

Don't forget to visit the companion website for this book at **www.ataglanceseries.com/nursing/learningdisability** to do some practice cases on these topics.

5 What is a learning disability?

Key components of learning disability are located in the interaction between the person, who may have significant deficits, and the community, but the person can and will cope in the right environment and with the right support

Support

Individual

Before 18 years old

IQ

Social competence

Environment

Introduction

In this chapter the term learning disability (LD) is defined. It will be shown that LD is identified by the presence of a significantly reduced ability to understand new or complex information (impaired intelligence), with a reduced ability to cope independently (impaired social functioning), and which occurred before 18 years of age. There is general agreement that 3–4/1000 of the general population will have a severe LD, and that 25–30/1000 of the general population will have a mild LD. It is important to emphasise that people with LD share a common humanity with fellow citizens in their communities, and in the wider society in which they live. Most of us desire love and a sense of connection with others; wish to be safe, to learn, to lead a meaningful life, to be free from ridicule and harm, to be healthy, and free from poverty, and in this respect people with LD are no different. All healthcare workers have a professional responsibility to bring about their inclusion into their communities by adhering at all times to a value base that respects them as fellow citizens. LD manifests in a number of different ways for each individual.

Intellectual profile

Fundamental to LD is a difficulty in learning and processing information. The following intellectual abilities may be impaired:

Verbal abilities

- Memory – including immediate recall of people, objects or events, and the ability to store and process information.

- Comprehension – understanding situations, knowing socially accepted norms, and being able to weigh up possible options.
- Language – vocabulary may be limited and some people may not understand words at all. Others may recognise words but struggle to understand more subtle meanings.
- Abstract thinking – may find it hard to separate themselves from the thing they are thinking about. Hypothetical situations are particularly difficult.

Non-verbal abilities

- Speed of processing – may take a long time to work out what is going on in a situation.
- Reasoning – shapes, patterns and numbers may be confusing and they can find it hard to put things in order.
- Coordination – there may be difficulty in coordinating movement or using fine motor skills.

Coping with everyday life

These difficulties in intellectual function can have an impact on a person's ability to cope with everyday life. This means that a person may have a range of difficulties that require support:

- Self care – including everything from getting up, washing, and dressing, through to going to bed.
- Domestic skills – looking after clothes, cooking and cleaning.
- Community living skills – getting out and about, managing simple social interactions, and using shops and public services, managing money.

Learning Disability Nursing at a Glance, First Edition. Edited by Bob Gates, Debra Fearns and Jo Welch. © 2015 John Wiley & Sons, Ltd. Published 2015 by John Wiley & Sons, Ltd.
Companion website: www.ataglanceseries.com/nursing/learningdisability

- Communication – getting on with people and being able to communicate needs and wishes.
- Work and leisure – using time purposefully, having fun and pursuing personal goals.

Behavioural phenotypes

Some people with LD have specific syndromes, and these may be associated with a particular profile of verbal and non-verbal abilities. For example, people who are on the autistic spectrum of conditions are characterised by specific difficulties with social communication and information processing. Information about specific syndromes is important in understanding and predicting possible manifestations of LD.

Additional needs

People with LD are more likely to have a range of additional health needs than does the general population. These are explored in subsequent chapters and are often referred to as co-morbidity of conditions.

Degrees of learning disability

For many years, LD has been divided into a number of categories to reflect its nature and extent. These range from 'borderline' through 'mild', 'moderate' and 'severe', to 'profound'. This represents one understanding of LD but there are others. This understanding uses the World Health Organisation classification system that defines the degree of disability according to how far an individual is from the normal distribution of IQ for the general population. Using this system, an individual who consistently scores more than two Standard Deviations (SD) on an IQ test, that is, a measured IQ of <70, is said to have LD. Individuals whose IQ is 50–69 are generally identified as having mild LD (F70); those with an IQ of 71–84 are said to be on the borderline of intellectual functioning; moderate LD (F71) is when the IQ is 35–49; the term severe learning disability (F72) is reserved for people whose IQ is 20–34; finally, the term profound learning disability (F73) refers to those with an IQ of <20. An alternative approach is based on a model of LD that sees it as an interaction between a person, the support they receive, and the environment they are located in. Each individual has a unique profile of LD that impacts on everyday life in different ways. There is a system for categorising the amount of support people need on four levels:

- Intermittent – this is time limited support at key times in life, such as loss of key relationships or transition.
- Limited – consistent need of support for specific tasks, such as employment training; still time limited.
- Extensive – regular long-term direct support in at least one setting.
- Pervasive – constant high-intensity support across all settings.

To this is added an assessment of the kind of environment a person needs, and the opportunities that are important for them to be healthy and achieve their personal goals. It is always important to remember that quality of life and relationships are very important to everyone whatever the degree of LD.

Definition of learning disability

Learning disability has been understood from a number of different theoretical perspectives. Three key perspectives are:

Sociological – From this perspective learning disability can be seen as deviance where learning disability might be seen as a subculture; distinct and different from other groups in society.

Medical – this focuses on the possibility that there is an underlying disease or pathology that might at some point be identified and understood, and treated as a medical condition.

Statistical – here it is assumed that any aspect of human behaviour can be measured, and will have a 'mean' and 'standard deviation'. In the case of LD there are two aspects of measurement: intelligence as measured by intelligence tests to arrive at an IQ, and adaptive behaviour – the ability to cope with the challenges of everyday life. People with a learning disability are defined as those who fall below a predefined level based on statistical means for the general population.

Summary

LD may be understood as an interaction between the person and the community. A person may have significant deficits but cope well in the right environment, and with the right support. But it should be remembered that minor difficulties can be massively disabling in a world where a person is isolated and unsupported. To conclude, in the UK all of these ideas have led to an accepted definition of LD which comprises three main components:

- significant lifelong difficulty in learning and understanding and,
- a significant difficulty in learning, and practising the skills needed to cope with everyday life, and
- that there is evidence that these difficulties started before 18 years of age.

6 Causes of learning disability

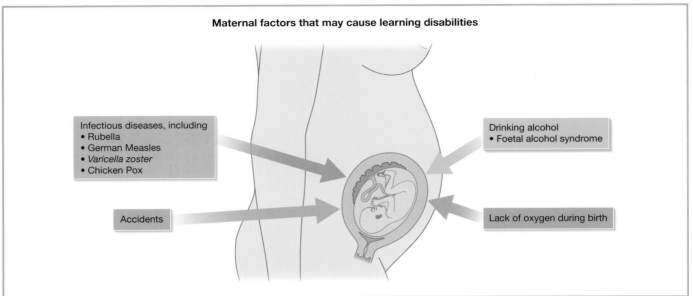

Maternal factors that may cause learning disabilities

Infectious diseases, including
- Rubella
- German Measles
- *Varicella zoster*
- Chicken Pox

Accidents

Drinking alcohol
- Foetal alcohol syndrome

Lack of oxygen during birth

Learning Disability Nursing at a Glance, First Edition. Edited by Bob Gates, Debra Fearns and Jo Welch. © 2015 John Wiley & Sons, Ltd. Published 2015 by John Wiley & Sons, Ltd.
Companion website: www.ataglanceseries.com/nursing/learningdisability

Maternal factors

Some infections acquired by the mother may be passed on to the unborn child through the placenta, and may lead to a learning disability in the child.

Rubella also known as 'German measles' is one infectious disease that can cause disability if a mother contracts it during the first three months of pregnancy. It affects the central nervous system in addition to the heart and blood vessels of the foetus. Infection in the first 8–10 weeks of pregnancy results in damage in up to 90% of surviving infants. Multiple defects are then common.

Frequency of congenital rubella following maternal infection is 50% during weeks 13–14. Severe malformations occur in virtually all foetuses infected before 12 weeks. If a woman contracts Rubella after 16 weeks of pregnancy, there is little risk of the foetus developing abnormalities. Rubella can be prevented by immunisation of all girls.

Varicella zoster, more commonly known as 'Chicken pox' poses a risk to the foetus if acquired during the first five months of pregnancy. Principal malformations include cataracts, microcephaly and learning disability. Infection with chickenpox during the first 28 weeks of pregnancy carries a risk that the foetus could develop a condition known as foetal varicella syndrome (FVS). This syndrome is rare. The risk of it occurring in the first 12 weeks of pregnancy is less than 1%. Between 13 and 20 weeks, the risk is 2%.

Foetal varicella syndrome can cause serious complications, including: scarring, eye defects, such as cataracts, shortened limbs and brain damage.

There are also other risks from catching chickenpox after week 20 of pregnancy. It is possible that the baby may be born prematurely (before week 37 of the pregnancy). In addition, if a pregnant woman is infected with chickenpox seven days before or seven days after giving birth, the newborn baby may develop a more serious type of chickenpox. In a few severe cases, this type of chickenpox can be fatal.

Neural tube defects: failure of the neural tube to fuse completely is linked to genetic factors, although these are usually due to multifactorial causes. A young maternal age and low socioeconomic status, and deficiency of folic acid vitamin are associated with neural tube defects.

Administration of multivitamin preparations containing folic acid during the first 6 weeks of pregnancy have resulted in a significant reduction in the incidence of new cases. New guidance also suggests that women trying to become pregnant should take folic acid in the months before getting pregnant. Pre-natal diagnosis is by ultrasound and measuring the level of alpha-fetoprotein in the amniotic fluid.

Foetal alcohol syndrome: Foetal alcohol syndrome (FAS) is the more severe end of a continuum of birth defects known as foetal alcohol spectrum disorders (FASDs).

Foetal alcohol effects (FAEs), otherwise known as alcohol-related birth defects (ARBDs), may represent the milder end of the spectrum. Other terms for conditions which come under the umbrella of FASD are alcohol-related neuro-developmental disorder (ARND) and partial foetal alcohol syndrome (pFAS). These are caused by maternal use of alcohol during pregnancy. There are three main characteristics of FAS:

- Typical facial abnormalities.
- Intrauterine growth restriction and failure to catch up.
- Neuro-developmental abnormalities causing learning disability, cognitive impairment and behavioural problems.

Risk factors: in the UK, NICE guidelines, the British Medical Association (BMA) guidance and the Royal College of Obstetricians and Gynaecologists (RCOG) statement concur that women should be advised to abstain from alcohol if possible in view of the uncertainty of risk, and in particular in the first three months due to the increased risk of miscarriage. If women choose to drink alcohol, they are advised to have no more than 1–2 units of alcohol no more than 1–2 times a week, as there is no evidence of harm at this level. They are also advised that binge drinking may harm the baby.

During and shortly after birth

A learning disability may result if the baby's oxygen supply is interrupted for a significant length of time, or if the baby is born significantly premature and becomes ill shortly after birth.

Some childhood infections can affect the brain, causing learning disability; the most common of these are *encephalitis* (inflammation of the brain) and *meningitis* which is an infection of the meninges (protective membranes) that surround the brain and spinal cord. The infection causes the meninges to become inflamed (swollen), which in some cases can damage the nerves and brain.

Social and environmental factors, such as poor housing conditions, poor diet and healthcare, malnutrition, lack of stimulation and child abuse may lead to learning disability.

Accidents: some babies who are severely injured in accidents will suffer permanent disability, and this may include learning disability.

Burns/scalds: of during the acute period of the burn there is serious disturbance of electrolyte metabolism, this can result in some brain damage.

7 Chromosomal disorders

Definition:
A chromosome is a thread-like structure of nucleic acids and protein found in the nucleus of most living cells, carrying genetic information in the form of genes. Humans have 22 pairs plus the two sex chromosomes (two X chromosomes in females, one X and one Y in males).

(a) Down's syndrome

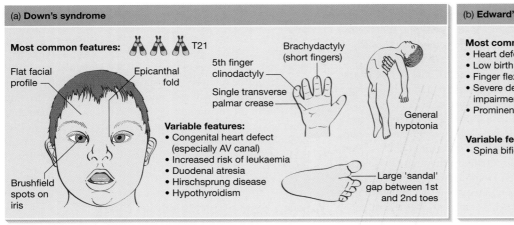

Most common features: T21

Flat facial profile

Epicanthal fold

5th finger clinodactyly

Brachydactyly (short fingers)

Single transverse palmar crease

General hypotonia

Brushfield spots on iris

Variable features:
- Congenital heart defect (especially AV canal)
- Increased risk of leukaemia
- Duodenal atresia
- Hirschsprung disease
- Hypothyroidism

Large 'sandal' gap between 1st and 2nd toes

(b) Edward's syndrome

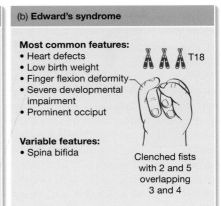

Most common features:
- Heart defects
- Low birth weight
- Finger flexion deformity
- Severe developmental impairment
- Prominent occiput

Variable features:
- Spina bifida

T18

Clenched fists with 2 and 5 overlapping 3 and 4

(c) Patau syndrome

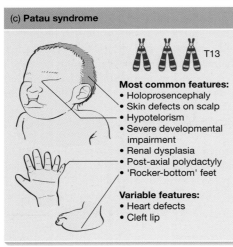

T13

Most common features:
- Holoprosencephaly
- Skin defects on scalp
- Hypotelorism
- Severe developmental impairment
- Renal dysplasia
- Post-axial polydactyly
- 'Rocker-bottom' feet

Variable features:
- Heart defects
- Cleft lip

(d) Prader–Willi

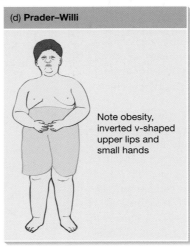

Note obesity, inverted v-shaped upper lips and small hands

(e) Klinefelter's syndrome

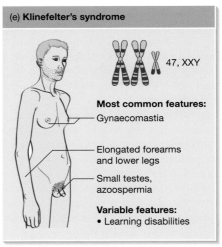

47, XXY

Most common features:
Gynaecomastia

Elongated forearms and lower legs

Small testes, azoospermia

Variable features:
- Learning disabilities

Source: Pritchard, D. & Korf, B. (2013) *Medical Genetics at a Glance*, 3rd edn. Reproduced with permission of Wiley.

Learning Disability Nursing at a Glance, First Edition. Edited by Bob Gates, Debra Fearns and Jo Welch. © 2015 John Wiley & Sons, Ltd. Published 2015 by John Wiley & Sons, Ltd.
Companion website: www.ataglanceseries.com/nursing/learningdisability

Chromosomal disorders

Chromosomes make up the genetic blueprint of every individual and normally each human has 46 chromosomes. Two of these chromosomes are the sex chromosomes, Y and Y. Chromosomes are composed of DNA (deoxyribonucleic acid) and therefore are the physical form in which our genes exist. The composition of the chromosomes for females is 46XX, while for males it is 46XY. Each half of the pair of chromosomes is inherited from each parent. Sometimes there can be an abnormality in an individual's chromosomes, and this may lead, in some cases, to learning disability.

Down's syndrome (trisomy 21)

The most well-known type of chromosome abnormality is Down's syndrome. Instead of having two no. 21 chromosomes, individuals affected by the condition have three. Down's syndrome is associated with impairment of cognitive ability and physical growth, as well as a particular set of facial characteristics. Heart defects are also common and are present at birth

Down's syndrome is not common, but the chances of having an affected baby increase as you get older. If a previous pregnancy has been affected by Down's syndrome, your risk is increased threefold.

The age factor

The risk of having a baby with Down's syndrome is:
- 1 in 1500 at age 20.
- 1 in 350 at age 35.
- 1 in 50 at age 43.

Common physical features of Down syndrome include *microgenia* (an abnormally small chin), an unusually round face, *macroglossia* (protruding/oversized tongue), almond-shaped eyes caused by an epicanthic fold of the eyelid, up slanting *palpebral fissures* (separation between upper and lower eyelids), shorter than normal limbs, a single transverse palmar crease, poor muscle tone and a larger than normal space between toes. People with Down's syndrome are also prone to other health issues, including thyroid issues, visual impairments, ear infections and hearing difficulties, increased risk of chest infections and early onset dementia.

Trisomy 13 (Patau syndrome)

Occurs in about 1 in 4000 to 1 in 10 000 live births with the risk increasing with maternal age. Affected babies have a profound degree of learning disability. Often infants die before their first birthday, with only 5% surviving beyond 3 years of age.

Trisomy 18 (Edward's syndrome)

Babies with Edward's syndrome grow slowly in the womb and have a low birth weight. Edward's syndrome can be identified by characteristic features, although the diagnosis must be confirmed with genetic tests. A third of babies born alive will die within a month of birth because of life-threatening medical problems.

Only 5–10% of babies with full Edward's syndrome survives beyond one year, and will live with severe disabilities.

Prader-Willi syndrome

Caused by deletions of chromosomes 15q, 11–13. Babies are generally full term, but small for gestational age. They fail to thrive and have severe feeding difficulties.

The syndrome typically causes low muscle tone with motor development delays, short stature if not treated with growth hormone, and incomplete sexual development. Most babies with Prader-Willi syndrome are floppy at birth with initial difficulties in feeding, but then in early childhood begin to show increased appetite which can lead to excessive eating and life-threatening obesity. They usually have a moderate degree of learning disability.

Klinefelter's syndrome

Klinefelter's syndrome (KS) occurs when males are born with an extra X chromosome. It is a genetic problem that only affects boys and men. It is a sex chromosome trisomy. Instead of being 46, XY, men or boys with KS are usually 47, XXY.

The condition affects sexual development and means that during puberty the normal male sexual characteristics do not develop fully. There is reduced facial and pubic hair, and some breast tissue may develop due to the lack of testosterone. It is not usually diagnosed until puberty.

Fragile X

Fragile X occurs due to changes on the X chromosome in a specific gene that makes a protein necessary for brain development. Boys are usually more severely affected than girls as they have only one X chromosome. Girls have a second X chromosome, which can compensate for problems with the faulty one.

The resulting learning disability can range from mild to severe learning disabilities. Some of the physical features include a relatively large head, a long face with prominent ears, largish jaw and double-jointedness.

Summary
- Chromosomes are made of DNA.
- Each contains genes in a linear order.
- Human body cells contain 46 chromosomes in 23 pairs – one of each pair inherited from each parent.
- Chromosome pairs 1–22 are called autosomes.
- The 23rd pair are called sex chromosomes: XX is female, XY is male.

Genetic disorders

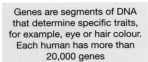

Genes are segments of DNA that determine specific traits, for example, eye or hair colour. Each human has more than 20,000 genes

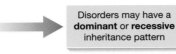

Disorders may have a **dominant** or **recessive** inheritance pattern

Dominant inheritance
A mutation only needs to be passed on from either the mother or the father

Recessive inheritance
Both parents must have a copy of the faulty gene (they are 'carriers' of the condition) in order to pass on the condition

Girl with karyotype 46,XX,del(5)(p15.2) showing Cri-du-chat syndrome

Note small head, widely spaced eyes, epicanthal folds, depressed nasal bridge, down-turned mouth

Man with karyotype 46,XY,del(17)(p11.2) showing Smith-Magenis syndrome

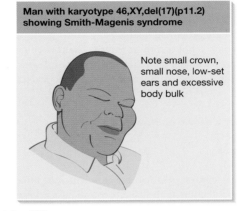

Note small crown, small nose, low-set ears and excessive body bulk

Source: Pritchard, D. & Korf, B. (2013) *Medical Genetics at a Glance*, 3rd edn. Reproduced with permission of Wiley.

Genetics and genetic disorders

What is genetics?

Genetics is the study of genes. Genes are segments of DNA (*deoxyribonucleic acid*) located on chromosomes. Genes are units inside a cell that control how living organisms inherit features from their ancestors, for example children usually look like their parents because they have inherited their parents' genes. Genetics tries to identify which features are inherited, and explain how these features pass from generation to generation.

The language used by DNA is called the genetic code.

Each cell in the body contains 23 pairs of chromosomes. These carry the genes inherited from parents. One of each pair of chromosomes is inherited from each parent, which means that with one exception, there are two copies of each gene in each cell.

The exception is with the X and Y sex chromosomes. These determine the sex of a baby. Babies with an X and a Y chromosome will be male (XY). Those without a Y chromosome, but two of the same kind of X chromosome, will be female (XX). This means that males only have one copy of each X chromosome gene.

The term 'genome' means all the genetic material carried in the body.

The human genome includes the complete set of genes contained in the human body. Apart from identical twins each individual's genome is unique.

What are genetic syndromes?

A syndrome is a disease or disorder that has *more than one identifying feature or symptom*. Each particular genetic syndrome will have many typical features, depending on which aspects of development are affected by the abnormal genes or chromosomes.

Angelman syndrome is a neuro-genetic disorder characterised by severe learning disability, sleep disturbance, seizures, jerky movements (especially hand-flapping), frequent laughter or smiling, and usually a happy demeanor.

Cri-du-chat syndrome, also known as **Lejeune's syndrome**, is a rare genetic disorder due to a missing part (deletion) of chromosome 5. Its name is a French term (*cat-cry* or *call of the cat*) referring to the characteristic cat-like cry of affected children. It is more common in girls than boys.

Symptoms include: feeding problems because of difficulty swallowing and sucking; low and poor growth; severe cognitive, speech, and motor delays; small head and jaw; wide eyes.

Rett syndrome: Rett syndrome is a genetic disorder that affects approximately 1 in 12 000 females (it is rarely seen in boys). It causes severe physical and mental disability that begins in early childhood.

Rett syndrome usually goes unnoticed for the first few months of the child's life, until major regression occurs at around one year of age, when children will lose acquired skills. People with Rett syndrome have profound and multiple physical and learning disabilities and are totally reliant on others for support throughout their lives.

Tay-Sachs disease is a rare disorder in which there is a progressive degeneration of all brain functions. Symptoms usually begin at around six months of age when their development begins to slow, and usually leads to death in early childhood. It affects girls and boys equally. It used to be common among Ashkenazi Jews – a group of Eastern European Jews – in whom about one in 25 people carry the gene. However, due to effective screening in this population, this condition is now rare.

Smith-Magenis syndrome is a rare genetic condition that may result in a moderate to severe learning disability. Someone with the syndrome is likely to need ongoing support and their support needs can be high.

Williams's syndrome is a genetic condition that will affect different individuals in different ways, but may cause a developmental delay or a learning disability. Physical therapy and speech and language therapy can help individuals with the condition

Phenylketonuria, (**PKU**) is a rare genetic condition that is present from birth. The body is unable to break down a substance called phenylalanine, which builds up in the blood and brain due to lack of an enzyme which breaks down certain amino acids. This can be detected shortly after birth and controlled through a diet low in phenylalanine, which can reduce the neurological damage associated with PKU.

If it goes undetected then severe learning disabilities can result. It is estimated to affect 1 in every 10 000 babies born in the UK and both sexes are affected equally. Screening is carried out by the heel prick test.

Summary

- Genes are units inside a cell that control how living organisms inherit features from their ancestors.
- Factors that influence the formation of genetic disorders include:
  - what genes are inherited
  - whether the gene for the condition is recessive or dominant.

9 Other causes of learning disability

There are a wide range of conditions that may lead to learning disability (LD). These include medical conditions (congenital and acquired), social and environmental factors. Aetiology is more easily established in cases of severe learning disability. Causes of LD can be attributed to insults that occur during the pre-natal, peri-natal and post-natal periods of the individual's life.

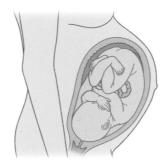 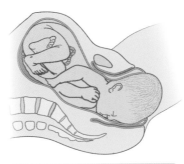 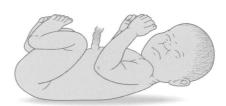

Pre-natal

- Chromosomal abnormalities: Down's syndrome
- Inborn errors of metabolism: PKU
- Genetic disorders: Fragile X, Rett syndrome
- Intrauterine infection: toxoplasmosis, rubella, herpes, CMV (TORCH)
- Intrauterine toxins: alcohol, narcotics, anti-epileptic drugs
- Recognisable syndromes: Soto's syndrome, tubular sclerosis
- Cerebral malformation: Agryia pachygyria
- Other: Duchenne's muscular dystrophy, congenital hypothyroidism

Peri-natal

- Birth asphyxia
- Neonatal meningo-encephalitis
- Maternal factors: ante-partum haemorrhage, pre-eclampsia
- Spontaneous pre-term delivery

Post-natal

- Infection: meningitis, encephalitis
- Hypoxic ischaemia: drowning, smothering
- Trauma: head injury, non-accidental injury
- Epileptic encephalopathies: West syndrome, Lennox Gastau syndrome

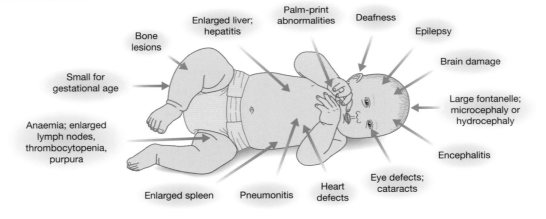

Bone lesions

Enlarged liver; hepatitis

Palm-print abnormalities

Deafness

Epilepsy

Brain damage

Small for gestational age

Large fontanelle; microcephaly or hydrocephaly

Anaemia; enlarged lymph nodes, thrombocytopenia, purpura

Encephalitis

Enlarged spleen

Pneumonitis

Heart defects

Eye defects; cataracts

Learning Disability Nursing at a Glance, First Edition. Edited by Bob Gates, Debra Fearns and Jo Welch. © 2015 John Wiley & Sons, Ltd. Published 2015 by John Wiley & Sons, Ltd.
Companion website: www.ataglanceseries.com/nursing/learningdisability

Intrauterine toxins

Drugs interfere with embryogenesis by exerting their pharmacological action on the developing foetal organs. The timing and dose of the drug, along with the efficiency of the mother's metabolism, placental transfer and susceptibility of the foetus will determine the degree of adversity.

Foetal alcohol spectrum disorder (FASD)

Excessive amounts of alcohol consumed during early pregnancy may lead to facial abnormalities, growth failure, microcephaly, skeletal and visceral abnormalities. Facial defects include micrognathia, hypoplasia of the mid face, beaking of the forehead, ear deformities and a small upturned nose. Major defects include cleft lip and palate, cardiac, ocular, limb and renal malformation. Convulsion and neonatal withdrawal symptoms may occur in the newborn.

Intrauterine infection

Maternal pre-natal infection acts by causing inflammatory lesions of the foetus and interferes with cell division. Certain infections are known to cause congenital defects, such as rubella, toxoplasmosis, herpes simplex, HIV, varicella and parovirus B19.

Rubella: high immunisation rates have led to reduced cases of congenital rubella syndrome.

Toxoplasmosis is an infection caused by the parasite *Toxoplasma gondii*, a microscopic single-cell organism that can be found in meat, cat faeces, the soil where cats defecate and unpasteurised goats' milk. The parasite can infect humans as well as birds and other warm blooded animals such as cats. Toxoplasmosis is only a risk to an unborn baby if caught for the first time during pregnancy or within a few weeks prior to conception. An unborn baby who contracts the disease will have congenital toxoplasmosis. The degree of risk to the foetus, and the damage caused, depends on when in pregnancy the mother acquired the infection.

Toxoplasmosis can potentially cause miscarriage, stillbirth or damage to the baby's brain and other organs, particularly the eyes. Most babies born with toxoplasmosis have no obvious damage at birth but will develop symptoms, typically eye damage, during childhood or even adulthood. A few may have more serious symptoms including blindness or brain damage.

Birth asphyxia

The syndrome associated with birth asphyxia is hypoxic ischaemic encephalopathy (HIE). HIE may be primary or secondary: primary occurs in utero, for example meconium aspiration, or it can occur after birth. It is a combination of hypoxia and ischemia that occurs simultaneously.

The severity of HIE is ascribed retrospectively to grades 1–3.

Grade 1: irritability, hyper-alert, mild hypotonia, poor sucking.

Grade 2: lethargy, seizures, marked abnormality of tone, tube feeding required.

Grade 3: coma, prolonged seizures, sever hypertonia, fails to maintain spontaneous respirations.

The severity of HIE is the most appropriate indicator of prognosis. Cerebral palsy, mental retardation, epilepsy, blindness, deafness hydrocephaly or microcephaly area all features of birth asphyxia. Specific learning difficulties, behavioural problems and clumsiness may not become evident until the child is older.

Birth injury

Injury to the baby may occur during labour or birth. Many injuries will be self-limiting and the infant will recover with no long-term deficits. There are many predisposing factors such as the shape and flexibility of the birth canal, presentation of the foetus, type of labour, delivery method: forceps, vacuum, that can contribute to injury – particularly injury to the head – and cause subdural haemorrhage.

Intracranial haemorrhage (ICH)

The five types of intracranial haemorrhage that occur in the infant are: subarachnoid, subdural, intraventricular, intracerebral and intracerebellar. Intraventricular is the most common type. Long-term outcomes are variable and range from no deficits occurring to serious neurological sequelae requiring lifelong treatment and care.

Neonatal sepsis

This is a generalised infection that is characterised by a proliferation of bacteria in the bloodstream commonly involving the meninges as opposed to bacteriaemia. It carries a high mortality rate. Long-term outcomes are dependent on response to treatment

Nursing considerations

Supportive care for the family is essential in helping them come to terms with their child's potential limitations and in accepting the diagnosis. This will include liaison with appropriate professionals, multidisciplinary discharge planning and coordination of ongoing care.

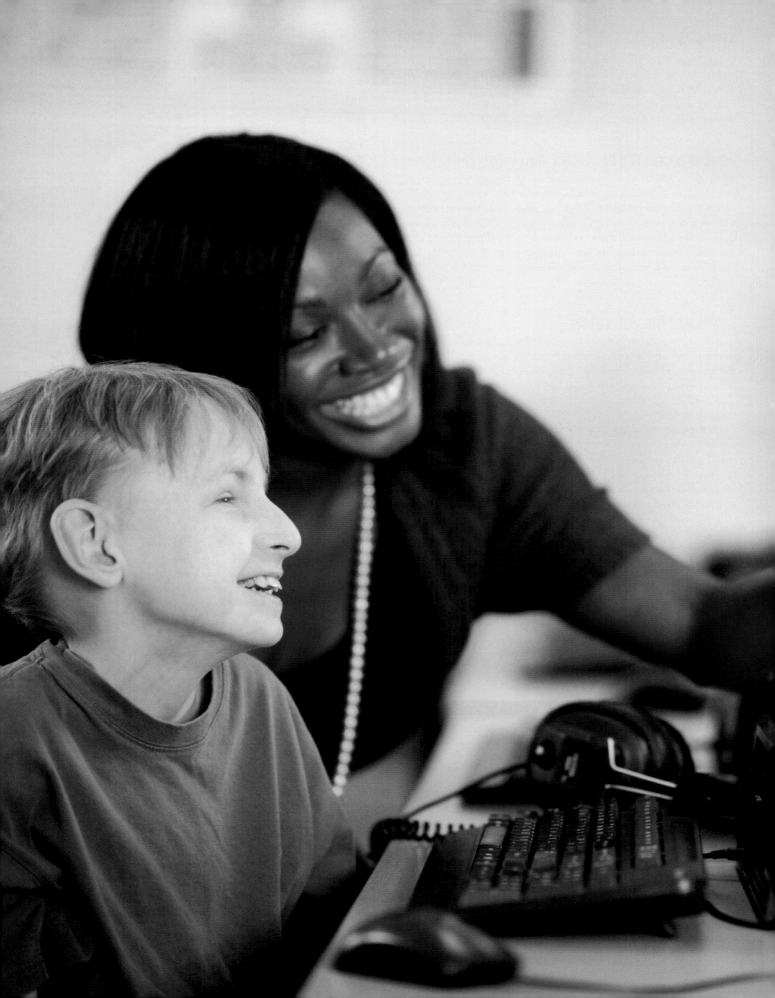

Childhood development

Part 3

Chapters

10 **Screening and genetics** 22
11 **Developmental milestones** 24
12 **Common childhood diseases** 26
13 **Developing communication** 28
14 **Learning through play** 30
15 **Education** 32
16 **Screening for autistic spectrum conditions** 34
17 **Safeguarding children** 36

 Don't forget to visit the companion website for this book at **www.ataglanceseries.com/nursing/learningdisability** to do some practice cases on these topics.

10 Screening and genetics

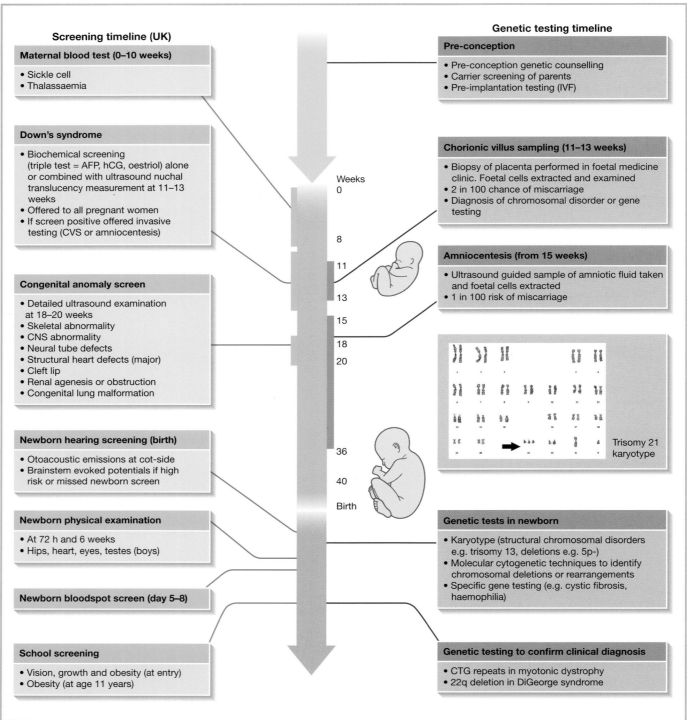

Screening timeline (UK)

Maternal blood test (0–10 weeks)
- Sickle cell
- Thalassaemia

Down's syndrome
- Biochemical screening (triple test = AFP, hCG, oestriol) alone or combined with ultrasound nuchal translucency measurement at 11–13 weeks
- Offered to all pregnant women
- If screen positive offered invasive testing (CVS or amniocentesis)

Congenital anomaly screen
- Detailed ultrasound examination at 18–20 weeks
- Skeletal abnormality
- CNS abnormality
- Neural tube defects
- Structural heart defects (major)
- Cleft lip
- Renal agenesis or obstruction
- Congenital lung malformation

Newborn hearing screening (birth)
- Otoacoustic emissions at cot-side
- Brainstem evoked potentials if high risk or missed newborn screen

Newborn physical examination
- At 72 h and 6 weeks
- Hips, heart, eyes, testes (boys)

Newborn bloodspot screen (day 5–8)

School screening
- Vision, growth and obesity (at entry)
- Obesity (at age 11 years)

Genetic testing timeline

Pre-conception
- Pre-conception genetic counselling
- Carrier screening of parents
- Pre-implantation testing (IVF)

Chorionic villus sampling (11–13 weeks)
- Biopsy of placenta performed in foetal medicine clinic. Foetal cells extracted and examined
- 2 in 100 chance of miscarriage
- Diagnosis of chromosomal disorder or gene testing

Amniocentesis (from 15 weeks)
- Ultrasound guided sample of amniotic fluid taken and foetal cells extracted
- 1 in 100 risk of miscarriage

Trisomy 21 karyotype

Genetic tests in newborn
- Karyotype (structural chromosomal disorders e.g. trisomy 13, deletions e.g. 5p-)
- Molecular cytogenetic techniques to identify chromosomal deletions or rearrangements
- Specific gene testing (e.g. cystic fibrosis, haemophilia)

Genetic testing to confirm clinical diagnosis
- CTG repeats in myotonic dystrophy
- 22q deletion in DiGeorge syndrome

Weeks 0, 8, 11, 13, 15, 18, 20, 36, 40, Birth

Learning Disability Nursing at a Glance, First Edition. Edited by Bob Gates, Debra Fearns and Jo Welch. © 2015 John Wiley & Sons, Ltd. Published 2015 by John Wiley & Sons, Ltd.
Companion website: www.ataglanceseries.com/nursing/learningdisability

Screening

Screening aims to identify unrecognised disease in apparently well people. Cost must be considered and balanced against that of treatment if the problem presents later. Conditions suitable for screening should:
• Be identifiable at a latent or early symptomatic stage.
• Be treatable.
• Have a better prognosis if treated early.

Screening of newborns and children in the UK is outlined opposite and in the box below. Further information is available at www.screening.nhs.uk/england.

Genetic disorders

Most disorders that are screened for in newborns have a genetic basis. Molecular genetic techniques are increasingly used to identify abnormal genes or chromosomes. It is vital that families receive appropriate counselling so that they understand the implications of an abnormal result. Genetic tests can be performed at various times:
• **Pre-implantation testing** is only available with in-vitro fertilisation techniques, but can allow screening prior to implantation.
• **Ante-natal genetic testing** via chorionic villus sampling or amniocentesis allows the possibility of termination of pregnancy. Some families choose to continue the pregnancy despite a positive result and this allows them time to come to terms with the diagnosis.
• **Newborn genetic testing** may be performed to confirm a clinical diagnosis (e.g. Down's syndrome or congenital myotonic dystrophy) or following a positive screening test (e.g. CF gene testing following an abnormal **IRT** result on the newborn blood spot screen).
• **Genetic testing of older children** may be needed to confirm a diagnosis presenting later in childhood (e.g. Fragile X or Duchenne muscular dystrophy). In general children must not be tested for adult-onset genetic disorders without their own informed consent unless it is going to alter their treatment during childhood.

Genetic inheritance

Many genetic disorders occur sporadically with no preceding family history or are multifactorial, with an environmental element (e.g. diabetes), but some single-gene disorders show a clear inheritance pattern:
• **Autosomal recessive**: both parents carry an abnormal copy of the gene (carrier): 25% of their children will inherit both abnormal genes and be affected; 50% of offspring inherit one abnormal gene and are themselves carriers and usually unaffected; 25% of offspring do not inherit either abnormal gene.
• **Autosomal dominant**: inheriting even a single copy of the abnormal gene from either parent means the child is affected. These conditions sometimes present earlier or more severely in successive generations (anticipation). Sometimes the effect of a gene mutation will depend on which parent it is inherited from (imprinting).
• **Sex-linked inheritance**: gene disorders on the X chromosome, usually only present in boys as the presence of a second normal X chromosome in girls prevents them being severely affected. Examples include haemophilia A and Fragile X syndrome.
• **Chromosomal disorders**: these are usually sporadic due to non-disjunction of chromosomes during meiosis (trisomy 21, 18 or 13) or due to rearrangement of major parts of the chromosome (translocations). In Turner's syndrome there is deletion of one X chromosome (45 XO). In some cases there is deletion of part of a chromosome, for example cri du chat syndrome (5p- deletion).

Screening for Down's syndrome

Down's syndrome affects 1 in 1000 live births (1 in 600 foetuses). There is an association with increased maternal age (1 in 880 at 30 years rising to 1 in 100 at age 40 years): 95% of cases are due to non-disjunction during meiosis and 3% to an unbalanced translocation; 1% are mosaics, with only a proportion of cells within the body having trisomy 21. About 55% of affected foetuses are detected ante-natally, through screening. In those diagnosed ante-natally, only 5% of couples choose to continue with the pregnancy. Antenatal screening involves measurement of AFP, hCG and oestriol (the 'triple' test) and other markers, with nuchal fold (subcutaneous tissue at back of the neck) thickness in the fetus. This gives a calculated risk, which if high may prompt diagnostic testing via chorionic villus sampling or amniocentesis.

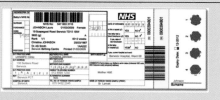

	Notes The midwife will collect bloodspots from the heel of every newborn baby on day 5-8 of life on to an absorbent card. These are analysed and also stored for further diagnostic tests if necessary
Congenital hypothyroidism	Screen detects high TSH level but will miss hypothyroidism secondary to pituitary dysfunction. Thyroid replacement allows normal development
Sickle cell disease	Universal screening to all pregnant women aims to identify at-risk couples. Newborn bloodspots are analysed by HPLC for all sickle cell variants
Phenylketonuria (PKU)	A phenylalanine assay has replaced the original 'Guthrie' test. Babies with PKU need urgent advice on starting a low-phenylalanine diet and long-term follow-up to prevent learning disability from phenylalanine metabolites
Cystic fibrosis (CF)	A high immunoreactive trypsin (**IRT**) on the newborn bloodspot is followed up with DNA testing for common CF mutations
Medium-chain acylcarnitine deficiency (MCAD)	A fatty acid oxidation defect that can lead to significant hypoglycaemia during periods of illness. Acylcarnitine abnormalities can be detected by tandem mass spectrometry. MCAD is a preventable cause of sudden death in infancy. Frequent feeds prevent the need for breakdown of fatty acids

11 Developmental milestones

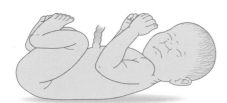

Growth and development begins before birth.
Development refers to an increase in capability or function.
Infants and children pass through predictable stages of development.

Four areas of development:

Gross motor development	Fine motor development
Social development	Speech and language development

Hearing and vision also need consideration.

When assessing developmental milestones:

Observe the child informally – young children may not co-operate with you

Listen to the parents – parental reporting of skills may be all you will get as the child may not want to talk to you

Prepare your environment – distraction will not be helpful

One task at time – young children have short attention spans

Be succinct in your assessment – know what you are assessing

Ask birth history – correct for prematurity until child is 2 years old

Development is an important indicator of the overall wellbeing of a child. Assessment of the developmental milestones is an integral part of all nursing and medical assessment of the child.

Developmental alert

As development is sequential and predictable, signs of developmental delay must be identified early.
Reassurance that normal development will occur is not appropriate.
Referral to a paediatrician should always be made if any of the following are present:

- Maternal concerns at any age.
- Regression of a previously acquired skill.
- Failure to smile by the age of 10 weeks.
- Hand preference, persistent primitive reflexes, squinting or no display of interest in people, toys, or noise at the age of six months.
- Not sitting up, no pincer grasp or not saying double syllable words such as ba-ba, ga-ga at the age of 10 months.
- Not able to say ma-ma, da-da (specific) by the age of 14 months.
- No independent walking, drooling and persistent mouthing and has less than six words at the age of 18 months.
- Unresponsive to name.
- Not stair climbing by the age of 2 years.
- Not able to combine 2–3 words by the age of 2½ (e.g. me outside, more milk).
- Unintelligible speech at the age of 4 years.

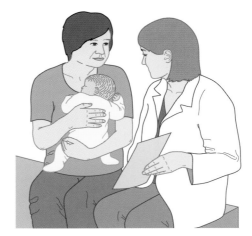

Learning Disability Nursing at a Glance, First Edition. Edited by Bob Gates, Debra Fearns and Jo Welch. © 2015 John Wiley & Sons, Ltd. Published 2015 by John Wiley & Sons, Ltd.
Companion website: www.ataglanceseries.com/nursing/learningdisability

Milestones of development

Age	Gross motor	Fine motor	Language	Social
Birth	Reflexive. Flexed posture. Complete head lag. Hand fisted.		Recognises parental voice. Makes throaty noises.	Shows interaction with people's faces. Gains satisfaction from being fed, held, rocking, cuddled.
One month-six weeks	Head control developing, raises head slightly from prone, pelvis flatter when in prone position. Curved back when sitting, needing adult support.	Shows eye coordination-eyes follow and focus vertically and horizontally.	Alert to sound	Smiles responsively.
4 months	Lifts head and shoulders when prone. Support weight on wrists and shifts weight to forearms when prone. No head lag. Intentional rolling over.	Holds a rattle and shakes it purposefully. Bring objects to mouth.	Vocalises. Coos.	Laughs out loud. Begins to respond to no. Enjoys sitting up. More interested in mother. Enjoys attention and can get bored if alone.
6 months	Arms extend supporting chest off surface when prone. Sits with self-propping. Stands with support. Rolls over well.	Reaches for objects and can transfer from hand to hand. Whole hand grasp.	Says 'Ma', 'Da'.	
7–8 months	Bounces and bears some weight when standing. May begin some form of mobility.	Finger feeds.	Makes talking sound in response to others. Double babble –'ma ma, da da'.	Self-contained play. Fear of strangers. Eye to eye contact when talking.
9 months	Gets into sitting position alone.	Immature pincer grasp.		Enjoys peek-a-boo, waves bye-bye.
10–12 months	Pulls to standing and stands holding on. Cruises around furniture. Stands and walks with one hand.	Mature pincer grasp. Turns pages in a book. Will hand a block/object to an adult. Can put balls in a box.	Begins to put two words together.	Points to get what they want. Responds to music. Shows fear, anger, affection, jealously, anxiety and sympathy. Increased attention span.
12–18 months	Walks independently. Stoops down to pick up objects.	Can build a tower of three or four blocks by the age 18 months.	Has 10 words of meaning. Imitates words. Points to objects named by adult.	Drinks from a cup. Spoon feeding self. Imitates adult behaviour. Follows directions and requests.
18–24 months	Walks up and down stairs. Steady gait. Kicks a ball in front of them. Rides a tricycle with walking action.	Scribbles with a pencil. Opens door handles. Build a tower of 4–6 blocks.	Able to link words together to make short sentences. Has 200–300 words. Refers to self by pronoun.	Imitates parents in domestic activities. Likes doll and ball games. Enjoys playing with other children. Short attention span. Spoon feeds self.
2–3 years	Throws objects overhead. Pedals tricycle. Walk backwards. Jumps.	Draws a circle. Drinks from a straw. Can string large beads.	900 word vocabulary. Talks incessantly. Can repeat 3 numbers.	Undress/dress self except buttons. Feeds self. Toilet trained by day.
4 years	Continuous movement going up and down stairs. Climbs well.	Draws a cross. Attempts to write letters.	1500 words, some number concept and asks many questions.	Buttons clothes, laces shoes. Imagination active.
5 years	Good motor control climbs and jumps well.	Draws a triangle and square. Prints first name.	2100 word vocabulary. Talks constantly.	Understands friendships. Power of reasoning.

12 Common childhood diseases

Chicken pox

Red itchy fluid-filled blisters which can be found anywhere on the body

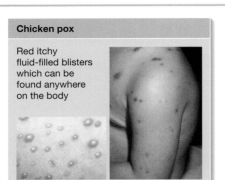

Hand foot and mouth disease

Blisters or spots with red edges develop in the mouth, on the tongue, on the palms of the hands, fingers and the soles of the feet

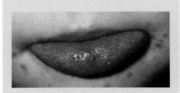

Rubella (German measles)

This tiny pink rash typically starts behind the ears but spreads all over the body

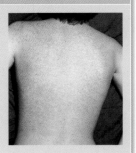

Molluscum contagiosum

Lumpy pink or whitish pearl-like spots, similar to small warts, on the face, arms, legs or trunk

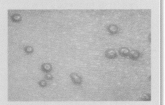

Mumps

Identifiable by swollen parotid glands below the ears

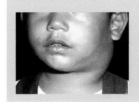

Measles

Typically starts in the mouth with small red spots with a bluish-white centre (Koplik spots). A few days later a widespread red raised blotchy rash appears

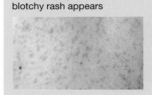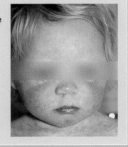

Impetigo

Pus-filled spots which crust, typically seen on the face and other exposed parts of the body

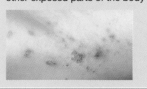

Scabies

The fine dark or silvery lines of the mite burrows are followed by a rash which is often apparent on the hands and feet of babies

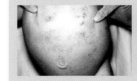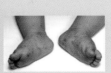

Learning Disability Nursing at a Glance, First Edition. Edited by Bob Gates, Debra Fearns and Jo Welch. © 2015 John Wiley & Sons, Ltd. Published 2015 by John Wiley & Sons, Ltd.
Companion website: www.ataglanceseries.com/nursing/learningdisability

Introduction

There are many childhood diseases which most children will catch one or more of as they are growing up. Many are relatively mild and cause little more than an irritable and fractious child for a couple of days. However, many also carry rare but severe complications. Infants and toddlers have not built up a robust immune system and are highly susceptible to these diseases which are easily spread from one child to another.

Spread

Infectious diseases are spread by several routes. For the diseases discussed here the following are relevant:
• Droplet – when the infected child coughs or sneezes, droplets containing the virus or bacteria are inhaled by a child. Droplets may also land on objects such as tables or door handles and can be transferred to a child.
• Direct contact – where one child comes into direct contact with the contaminant, such as the fluid from pustules.
• Faeces – some infectious diseases are present in the child's faecal matter and care must be taken to prevent spread via this route.
Disease can be spread by other routes including from a mother to her unborn child; from animals bites or faeces; by insect bites or from contaminated food.

Incubation period

The incubation period refers to the amount of time that elapses from first exposure to the pathogen to when the first signs and symptoms are visible. This is the time when the incoming pathogens multiply enough in the new recipient to produce signs of the disease. Each childhood disease has a different incubation period.

Contagious period

This is the length of time that the child may pass the infection to another person. Often in childhood diseases the child is contagious before the first visible signs are apparent, therefore childhood diseases are easily and unavoidably spread.

Diseases

Chicken pox (Varicella)

Generally a mild disease caused by the varicella zoster virus. It is easily spread by droplet or direct contact with the fluid from the pustules. Chicken pox has an incubation period of between 10 and 20 days and children are contagious from a few days before the first spot appears until the last spot has crusted over. The spots are very itchy and combined with a pyrexia makes children irritable, they may have anything from just a few spots to being covered in them. There is no specific treatment.

Measles/Mumps/Rubella

Due to the introduction of the measles, mumps and rubella (MMR) vaccine, these once common childhood diseases are now rarely seen, although outbreaks do occur in areas of poor uptake of the vaccine. They are all caused by a virus and spread by the droplet route.

Children with measles have a pyrexia and harsh cough along with the rash; the incubation period is 10 to 12 days and children are contagious from 4 days prior to the rash developing until 4 days after it has disappeared.

Mumps is characterised not only by the facial swelling but may be accompanied by a headache, joint pain and pyrexia. The incubation period is anything from 12 to 25 days. Children can be contagious from a couple of days before symptoms appear to about 5 days after the swelling subsides.

Rubella tends to be a mild disease with an incubation period of 2 to 3 weeks and children are contagious up to 1 week before and 4 days after the rash. There is no specific treatment for any of these diseases, although symptoms can be managed accordingly.

Hand, foot and mouth

A mild viral infection affecting younger children, which starts with a pyrexia and sore throat and is followed by spots in the mouth which spread primarily but not exclusively to the hands and the feet. The incubation period is 3 to 5 days but children may be infectious for some weeks afterwards as the virus is excreted in faeces. Good hygiene is therefore imperative.

Scabies

Scabies is caused by a tiny mite and spread by direct skin to skin contact, such as holding hands with an infected person. The mite burrows into the skin, causes intense itching and is followed by a blotchy rash. Symptoms can take 2 to 6 weeks to develop after being infected and treatment is with an insecticide cream.

Impetigo

A common bacterial infection of the skin, primary impetigo affects healthy skin; secondary impetigo affects skin already damaged for example by eczema. The rash typically develops 4 days after infection and children remain contagious until 24 hours after starting antibiotic treatment.

Molloscum contagiosum

A common vial condition which is spread by direct skin contact, the small mollusca (warts) tend to develop in clusters 2 to 8 weeks after being infected with the virus. Each molluscum can last for 6 to 12 weeks and it can take 12 to 18 months to finally clear up. No specific treatment.

Complications

Whilst generally mild, any of the rashes may become infected requiring further treatment with antibiotics; more serious complications are rare. However chicken pox, mumps and measles may cause viral encephalitis or meningitis and rubella can cause complications for an unborn baby such as deafness or congenital heart disease.

13 Developing communication

Developing communication is more than learning to speak. It is about learning to understand what people are trying to communicate to us.

- Language is the meaning of the words and putting those words together to make meaningful sentences
- Speech is the verbal means of communicating

Parts of language

Receptive language	Understanding of what is said to us
Expressive language	Use of language to communicate
Speech	Production of sounds
Phonology	Consonants and vowels that make up language
Syntax	The way that words make up a sentence
Grammar	The way parts of words make up a sentence
Morphology	Changes at word level to convey specific meaning
Semantics	Meaning of sentences and words
Pragmatics	Use of language in social situations
Prosody	Rhythm/stress of speech

How communication develops

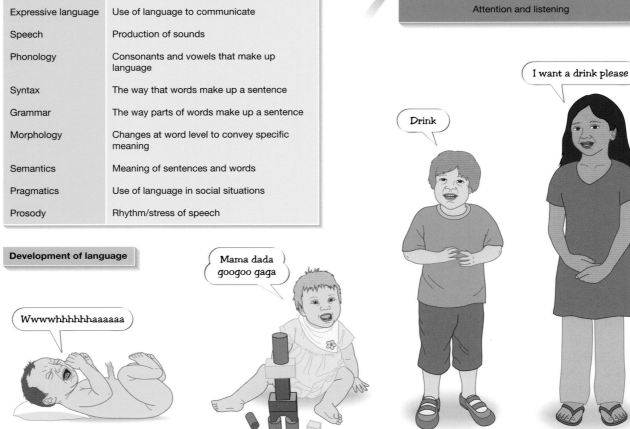

Development of language

This chapter briefly covers the development of communication.

Children start learning about communication before they are born. Within a few weeks they are watching adult's faces, experimenting with mouth movements and learning that making noises is a way to get their needs met.

The figure above shows the development of communication from birth, with developing speech sounds and perfecting speech as the final aspect of learning to communicate.

7% of speech is the words we speak; the other 93% is how we say the words, the facial expression we use, body language, meaning and context, (Mehrabian, 1971).

Attention and listening

Children learn by 12 months old to direct an adult's attention to what they want. This is a skill that is learnt through experience that when they cry they get their needs met, for example food, nappy changed, cuddle and so on. They also recognise their own name. As they develop further a child will be able to direct another person's attention to an object, this is known as joint attention.

If a child does not make eye contact, and has not developed joint attention, this could be an indication that there is a communication difficulty. A child not responding to their name, noises and not developing language could be an indication of a hearing impairment.

Symbolic play

Children learn many skills through symbolic play. Symbolic play is the ability of children to use objects, actions or ideas to represent other objects, actions or ideas as they play. Pretending to have a tea party with teddy bears, make believe shopping or pretending to make a phone call are all examples of symbolic play. An early example of symbolic play would be a child making noise with their baby toys by banging them or shaking them.

Psychologists look for examples of symbolic play in young children as a lack of this type of play skill could indicate Autistic Spectrum Disorder.

Understanding (receptive language)

Receptive language develops from the very simple one keyword level understanding up to reading body language and listening to the way others say things. Difficulties with receptive language can show in many ways, children may not reach their milestones as quickly as other children and they get older they may not learn the rules of using language like other children do. Sometimes a child will be delayed and may catch up with their peers and sometimes they may have a communication disorder with an underlying cause which means they may not catch up.

• By 12 months old a child begins to recognise common words such as daddy and cup.

• By 18 months a child will begin to understand simple instructions like 'kick ball'.

The table above explains the different parts of language we learn to understand.

Expressive language

Babies quickly learn to express a range of emotions and can request things to get their needs met. Through a range of non-verbal strategies babies quickly learn that humans communicate through social interaction.

• By 6 months old a baby is beginning to experiment with sounds and have different cries that mean different things.

• By 12 months old a child begins to string sounds and make noises to gain the adult's attention.

• By 3 years old most people can understand what the child is saying as the majority of speech sounds are developed.

Social communication

As humans we do not use communication just to get our needs met but also to socialise, make friends and form relationships. Alongside learning how to ask for things and listen to instructions, children learn to interact for pleasure. A child that avoids communicating other than to get their needs met may be showing signs of a communication difficulty.

• By 18 months old a child is beginning to learn turn taking and non-verbal gestures by copying adult behaviours.

• By 3 years old a child has developed play skills and begins learning to share.

Bilingualism

Language is learnt best before the age of 10. After this it becomes more difficult to remember the rules that make another language. Bilingual children may have a quiet period where they are processing all the information in the languages they are learning. This does not indicate a communication difficulty. A communication difficulty in a bilingual child will be apparent in all the languages the child speaks, not just one of them.

14 Learning through play

Introduction

The importance of play to a child cannot be underestimated. It is an essential requirement for physical and emotional development and wellbeing, and could be described as the universal language of all children.

Children's ability to communicate through play can be identified from infancy. When being sung to and played with by their parents, carers and significant people in their world, they begin to develop attachments, respond to stimulus and learn about the world around them.

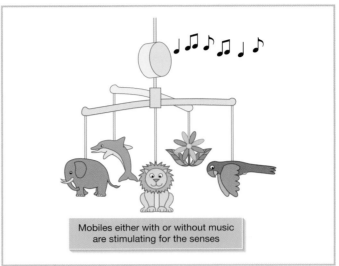

Mobiles either with or without music are stimulating for the senses

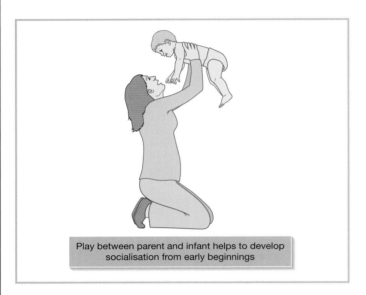

Play between parent and infant helps to develop socialisation from early beginnings

Resources required for play can be simple and inexpensive, beginning with being sung to and shown actions to rhymes when an infant and young child. Children under the age of 5 are particularly dependent on their senses of sight, touch and hearing when learning about their environment, this is evident when observing infants reaching for objects shown to them, or responding to music or toys that rattle. Sensory play continues to be comforting for older children with complex needs who may have some form of sensory deprivation but enjoy the stimulus of distraction suitable for their developmental needs. For example, play involving sounds, music and toys with different sensations related to touch enhance the world of children who may be visually impaired.

As a child grows, their dexterity skills develop and they master play though more complex activities, such as building blocks, water and sand play and creative activities such as drawing and painting. The medium of art is used therapeutically as a means of helping children to express themselves, especially if they have experienced situations that have caused them distress. Play is used widely in the therapeutic environment as a means of teaching children about what is likely to happen to them in relation to treatment; it is also used as a means of distraction from situations that may be causing them physical or emotional distress.

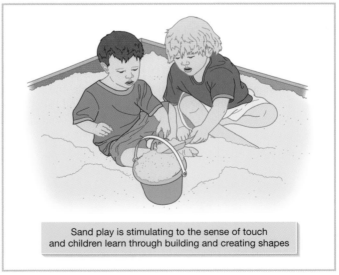

Sand play is stimulating to the sense of touch and children learn through building and creating shapes

Adults must be mindful of ensuring safety as children learn about their environment, through play. They also learn by copying the activities of adults. Young children, once mobile, will seek out objects for entertainment around them, and these may be hazardous Adults responsible for the child must not only provide age and developmentally appropriate play facilities but must also provide a safe and secure

Learning Disability Nursing at a Glance, First Edition. Edited by Bob Gates, Debra Fearns and Jo Welch. © 2015 John Wiley & Sons, Ltd. Published 2015 by John Wiley & Sons, Ltd.
Companion website: www.ataglanceseries.com/nursing/learningdisability

environment free from household dangers such as cleaning fluids, sharp objects and objects that could cause injury such as burns. While play involving water is often a popular and exciting environment for children of all ages and ability, adult supervision is essential in order to avoid injury. Water is important for encouraging assisted play with children who have disability, this is due to the lack of physical restriction and weightless sensation that a swimming pool can provide.

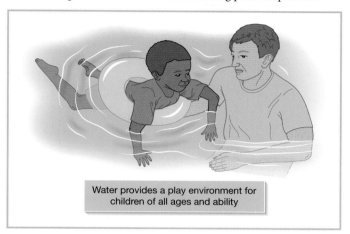

Water provides a play environment for children of all ages and ability

Children use play to socialise and integrate with their peers. Children under the age of 5 tend to play alongside each other rather than engage in collaborative play, but while playing they continue to communicate and discuss the play being engaged in.

Later, children develop the ability for imaginary play and this may often involve a group of children. By playing together children learn the skills of negotiation, inclusion, sharing and organisation; leadership skills can start to be identified while watching a group of children play. Earlier, play was described as the universal language of children, next time you are on holiday abroad observe how children overcome the barrier of language by engaging in play in swimming pools or taking part in a game of football on the beach.

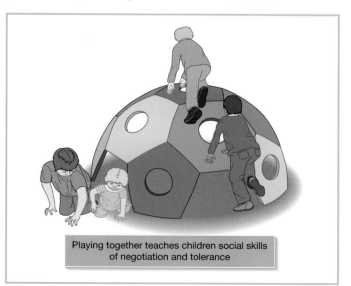

Playing together teaches children social skills of negotiation and tolerance

More recently technology games have become a familiar medium for play with older children, but adults should be mindful to encourage interaction with peers rather than play that lends itself to isolation in order that necessary life skills can continue to develop.

As children enter adolescence, play tends to become more formalised and complex in nature. This could take the form of team games or organised sport. Games that require an ability to consider complex rules and strategy lend themselves to the adolescent age group, for example football, tennis, chess. Play that involves teams or clubs teaches older children the importance of peer support and responsibility. A sense of belonging can be established and the emotional benefits of physical activity are considerable, this is an important consideration during the developmental period of adolescence.

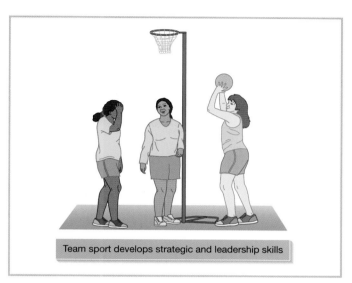

Team sport develops strategic and leadership skills

In order for all children to reach their full, individual potential it is essential that play is encouraged, engaged with and promoted in all environments where children live, learn and visit. Disability must never be a barrier to the universal language of play, as all children are able to develop and enjoy a sense of achievement through this essential activity.

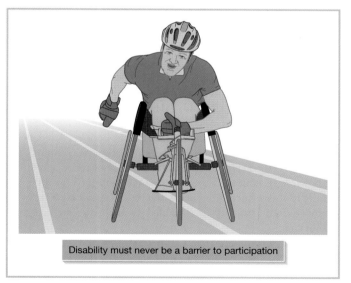

Disability must never be a barrier to participation

Summary
- Play is a fundamental requirement for a child's physical and emotional growth and wellbeing.
- Play is essential in helping children develop communication skills.
- Play enables children to negotiate friendships, and tolerance and respect.

15 # Education

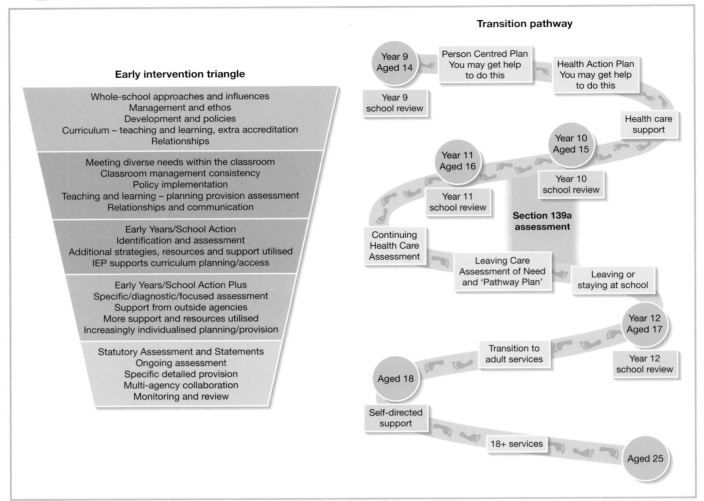

Early intervention triangle

Whole-school approaches and influences
Management and ethos
Development and policies
Curriculum – teaching and learning, extra accreditation
Relationships

Meeting diverse needs within the classroom
Classroom management consistency
Policy implementation
Teaching and learning – planning provision assessment
Relationships and communication

Early Years/School Action
Identification and assessment
Additional strategies, resources and support utilised
IEP supports curriculum planning/access

Early Years/School Action Plus
Specific/diagnostic/focused assessment
Support from outside agencies
More support and resources utilised
Increasingly individualised planning/provision

Statutory Assessment and Statements
Ongoing assessment
Specific detailed provision
Multi-agency collaboration
Monitoring and review

Transition pathway

Year 9 Aged 14
Person Centred Plan You may get help to do this
Health Action Plan You may get help to do this
Year 9 school review
Health care support
Year 10 Aged 15
Year 11 Aged 16
Year 10 school review
Year 11 school review
Section 139a assessment
Continuing Health Care Assessment
Leaving Care Assessment of Need and 'Pathway Plan'
Leaving or staying at school
Year 12 Aged 17
Transition to adult services
Year 12 school review
Aged 18
Self-directed support
18+ services
Aged 25

English children with Special Educational Needs (SEN) associated with learning disabilities are twice as likely as their peers to live in poor households (IHaL, 2012). In 2003/4, 27% of 13–14-year-old adolescents with mild to moderate learning disabilities who were attending mainstream school reported being bullied at least weekly (compared to 13% of children without SEN).

The special educational needs (SEN) code of practice requires schools, early education providers, local authorities and those who help them (including health and social services) to provide reasonable adjustments for disabled pupils. This code recommends that:
• special educational provision is matched to children's needs
• schools and LEAs embrace a graduated approach through School Action and School Action Plus and Early Years Action and Early Years Action Plus in early education settings.
All students with a statement of special educational needs (SEN) who are likely to leave school to move on to post-16 education and training are entitled to a Section 139a Learning Difficulty Assessment (LDA). This is a written report of the young person's educational or training needs and the provisions required to meet them. It is to help the young person, their parents and Children's Services staff to:
• identify and agree the most suitable post-16 learning provider;
• ensure that their needs are fully considered when matching a placement to meeting their individual needs;
• create the support the young person needs to achieve new goals in life;
• provide a plan that cover the young person up to the age of 25.

Definition of learning difficulties (for the purpose of education)

A young person has a learning purposes if:
• he/she has a significantly greater purposes in learning than the majority of persons of his age, or
• he/she has a disability which either prevents or hinders them from making use of facilities of a kind generally provided by institutions providing post-16 education or training.
Learning difficulty is the term used in legislation while 'learners with learning difficulties and/or disabilities' is a deliberately wide

Learning Disability Nursing at a Glance, First Edition. Edited by Bob Gates, Debra Fearns and Jo Welch. © 2015 John Wiley & Sons, Ltd. Published 2015 by John Wiley & Sons, Ltd.
Companion website: www.ataglanceseries.com/nursing/learningdisability

definition in common usage in the further education (FE) system, and includes people with mental health difficulties, autistic spectrum conditions, dyslexia, attention deficit hyperactivity disorder, behavioural emotional or social disorders, physical, sensory and cognitive impairments and other identified and non-identified difficulties in learning, which would include those with a learning disability.

From September 2012, schools and local authorities also have a duty to provide auxiliary aids and services to disabled pupils. This is to support inclusive education, which is a process by which a school attempts to respond to all pupils as individuals by reconsidering and restructuring its curricular organisation and provision and allocating resources to enhance equality of opportunity. This process enables the school to build capacity to accept all pupils from the locality who may wish to attend in order to reduce the need to exclude pupils due to their different abilities.

In order to identify the issues and be able to support issues in learning and continuing to support children with Special Educational Needs there is a 'statementing' process. To be able to undertake this thoroughly, inclusion philosophy needs schools to have a 'can do' attitude, to be creative in a 'think outside the box' way to meet the needs of children in line with the policy. An educationally inclusive school is one in which the teaching and learning, achievements, attitudes and wellbeing of every young person matters (OfSTED, 2002).

Identifying special educational needs

Most children who have a learning disability will have this diagnosis at birth, though some may not. Most, however, are evident by the age of 3 and therefore prior to school age. Each and every child is different and so are their educational needs, this will be dependent on their health and the complexities of these needs. These can be managed and discussed with the Special Needs Coordinator (SENCO). They are charged with working alongside the parent/carer and child to work out exactly what kind of extra support they may require. This may be anything from teaching methods to support in the classroom. They are also able to ask for help to support from external agencies, such as speech and language therapy or occupational therapy.

The SENCO is there to work with the school and the governing bodies in strategic development of the SEN policy and provision in order to raise the achievement of children with SEN. They have day to day responsibility for the operation of the SEN policy and coordination of the provision made for individual children with SEN, working closely with staff, parents, carers and other agencies. The SENCO also provides related professional guidance to colleagues with the aim of securing high quality teaching for children with SEN.

Legislation
Statutes
DfES: National Curriculum 2000
DfES: The Education Act 1996
DfES: SEN and Disability Act 2001 (amended 2005)
DCSF: The Children Act 2004

Statutory guidance
DfES: SEN Code of Practice
DfES: SEN Toolkit
DRC: DDA Part 4: Code of Practice 1995

DfES: Inclusive Schooling, Children with SEN 2001
DfES: Accessible Schools 2002
DfES: Access to Education for Children and Young People with Medical Needs 2000
DoH: Framework for the Assessment of Children in Need 2000
DfES: Removing Barriers to Achievement, The Government's Strategy for SEN 2004
DCSF: Every Child Matters: Change for Children 2004

The Children and Families Bill (currently in Parliament) will bring radical changes to the special educational needs (SEN) framework, this will look at a 0–25 Code of Practice. The Bill proposes replacing SEN statements (for schools) and Learning Difficulty Assessments (for young people in further education and training) with a single 0–25 Education, Health and Care Plan and aims to:
• give young people with special educational needs in further education and training aged 16–25 rights and protections comparable to those in school;
• require local authorities and local health services to plan and commission education, health and social care services jointly;
• require local authorities to publish in one place a clear and easy to understand 'local offer' of education, health and social care services to support children and young people with SEN and their families;
• require cooperation between local authorities and a wide range of partners, including schools, academies, colleges, other local authorities and services responsible for providing health and social care;
• require local authorities to consult with children and young people with SEN and their parents in reviewing special educational provision and social care provision;
• introduce a streamlined process for assessing the needs of those with more severe and complex needs, integrating education, health and care services and involving children, young people and their parents;
• replace statements and Learning Difficulty Assessments with a new 0–25 Education, Health and Care Plan, which will coordinate the support for children and young people and focus on desired outcomes including, as they get older, preparation for adulthood;
• encourage parents and young people to consider mediation to resolve disagreements before they register a Tribunal appeal;
• give parents and young people with an Education, Health and Care Plan the right to a personal budget for their support.

Changes from the SEN Code of Practice 2001
The main changes from the SEN Code of Practice (2001), to reflect the new legislation, are:
• The Code of Practice (2014) covers the 0–25 age range.
• There is a clearer focus on the views of children and young people and on their role in decision-making.
• It includes guidance on the joint planning and commissioning of services to ensure close cooperation between education, health services and social care.
• For children and young people with more complex needs, a coordinated assessment process and the new 0–25 Education, Health and Care Plan (EHC plan) replace statements and Learning Difficulty Assessments (LDAs).
• There is new guidance on the support pupils and students should receive in education and training settings.
• There is a greater focus on support that enables those with SEN to succeed in their education and make a successful transition to adulthood.

Screening for autistic spectrum conditions

16

Box A. Key actions recommended by The Improving Health and Lives: Learning Disabilities Observatory (2012).
This outlines key actions that all NHS Trusts and health services need to consider when implementing reasonable adjustments.

1	Ensure that people with learning disabilities and ASC are easily identified in records systems.
2	Foster a culture in which everyone understands reasonable adjustments and how they can help everyone when applied in a timely and appropriate manner.
3	Have a policy on accessible information and review coverage and use on a regular basis.
4	Promote the involvement of family carers in the healthcare of people with learning disabilities.
5	Continuously monitor how well the Mental Capacity Act 2006 is being implemented.
6	Develop clear and widely used protocols for service delivery and, where applicable, discharge arrangements that take account of the additional support needs of people with learning disabilities.
7	Ensure that people with learning disabilities and their family carers can influence what happens within the organisation at all levels.

Box B. Autistic Spectrum Criteria belonging to the DSM-V

The DSM-V Autistic Spectrum Conditions Criteria
• Onset before 3 years old   • At least six from the following (at least two from category 1):

1. Qualitative impairment in social interaction	2. Qualitative impairments in communication	3. Restricted, repetitive and stereotyped patterns of behaviour, interests and activities
• Marked impairment in the use of non-verbal behaviours such as eye contact, facial expression, body posture,etc. • Failure to develop peer relationships appropriate to developmental level • Lack of spontaneity in seeking to share enjoyment, interests with others • Lack of social reciprocity	• Delay or lack of spoken language with no compensatory non-verbal communication • In those with speech, impairment in the ability to initiate or sustain conversation • Stereotypical/receptive/idiosyncratic language • Lack of spontaneous and varied pretend play	• Preoccupation with one or more restricted interests that is unusual in intensity or focus • Inflexible adherence to routines or rituals • Stereotyped and repetitive movements • Preoccupation with parts of objects • Social play

Learning Disability Nursing at a Glance, First Edition. Edited by Bob Gates, Debra Fearns and Jo Welch. © 2015 John Wiley & Sons, Ltd. Published 2015 by John Wiley & Sons, Ltd.
Companion website: www.ataglanceseries.com/nursing/learningdisability

Screening for Autistic Spectrum Conditions (ASC)

In recent years, the number of children and adults with Autistic Spectrum Conditions (ASC) has growing significantly. There may be a number a reasons for this; however, the impact of improved screening and diagnostic procedures upon these figures are clear. Not only have the diagnostic tools and assessment formats become more sophisticated, the procedures of how to obtain a diagnosis and relevant services is becoming more accessible for people with ASC and their parents and carers.

The Autism Act (DoH, 2009) and subsequent Autism Strategy – Fulfilling and Rewarding Lives (DoH, 2010), highlight the need for screening procedures to be more efficient and the consequential access to services to be less problematic. The Autism Strategy calls for existing services to make *reasonable adjustments* or for new services to be set up meet the needs of people with ASC.

Many services in the UK are meeting the requirements of the Autism Strategy in different ways: there are a growing number of autism clinics being developed to assess and diagnose people with Autistic Spectrum Conditions, many of these clinics are attached to newly developed autism teams, which consist of a variety of disciplines including housing officers, social workers, parents, psychiatrists, psychologists and nurses who can act quickly to ensure a person with a new ASC diagnosis has access to appropriate health and social care services.

Diagnosis

The Diagnostic and Statistical Manual of Mental Disorders is widely regarded as the standard for diagnosis and would be in use in many of the clinics mentioned above by the person designated to diagnose, normally a psychiatrist or a clinical psychologist. However, it is important to note that the DSM-IV or similar used is not a checklist for diagnosis, but more a useful reference point. The (fifth) edition of the Diagnostic and Statistical Manual of Mental Disorders (DSM), DSM-5 was published in May 2013.

In children services, this checklist will often be completed by the health visitor or a GP, in adult services very often a learning disability nurse would apply this in liaison with a clinical psychologist. Regardless of who is using this, it is important that it is used as a discourse of information gathered via interviews and observations.

The three main groupings in Box B above are often referred to as the 'Triad of Impairment' and help to categorize elements of behaviour which can be attributed to Autism Spectrum Conditions.

However, within the changes made in the DSM-V. the Triad of Impairment will be reduced to two main areas:

1 Social communication and interaction.
2 Restricted, repetitive patterns of behaviour, interests, or activities.
(The National Autistic Society, 2012)

Additionally, sensory behaviours will be included in the criteria for the first time, under restricted, repetitive patterns of behaviour descriptors. There is an ever growing body of research analysing the hypersensitivities that people with ASC experience to some sounds, smells and visuals, more is written about this in Chapter 24.

Another change is that the DSM will no longer give a specific diagnosis; that is the current terms used in the DSM-V which are autistic disorder, Asperger's disorder, childhood disintegrative disorder and PDD-NOS (pervasive developmental disorder not otherwise specified) have been removed from DSM 5.

The proposals mean that when people go for a diagnosis in future, instead of receiving a diagnosis of one of these disorders, they would be given a diagnosis of Autism Spectrum Condition.

The National Autistic Society (2012) has collated information from those people with Asperger's in particular, as they appear to be unhappy that this term will no longer be used in the DSM.

17 Safeguarding children

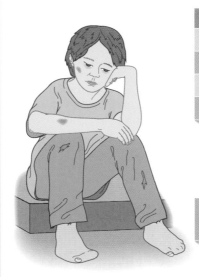

Safeguarding children is defined as:

- Protecting children from maltreatment

- Preventing impairment of children's health and development

- Enabling children to reach their full potential by providing a secure environment and safe effective care

- Undertaking roles to ensure children have the optimum opportunity to enter adulthood successfully

Children and young people with a disability are three times more likely to be abused or neglected than their non-disabled peers

Child protection is every nurse's responsibility and a nurse has an absolute duty to safeguard and protect children and young people. If there is any suspicion of child abuse then the child should be immediately referred to the child protection team.

Categories of child abuse

Physical abuse	Neglect	Emotional abuse	Sexual abuse
Physical abuse may involve: hitting, shaking, burning, scalding, throwing, poisoning, drowning, suffocating or other physical harm to the child. It also includes fabricated symptoms or deliberately induced illness by the parent/carer	Neglect is the persistent failure to meet the child's basic physical and/psychological needs resulting in serious impairment to the child's health and/or development. Ante-natally, this can include maternal substance abuse. Included in this category are parental failure to provide adequate food, clothing, shelter and protection from harm	Emotional abuse is the persistent emotional ill-treatment of a child such as to cause severe effects on their emotional development. This may include telling the child they are worthless, unloved, unwanted. Overprotection and prevention of the child from participation in normal social activities are included, as is witnessing the ill-treatment of another	Sexual abuse is the forcing or enticing of a child or young person to participate in sexual activities. This includes prostitution. The activities may involve physical contact – penetrative and non-penetrative acts – and non-contact activities such as encouraging children to behave in a sexually inappropriate manner, watching sexually explicit acts/material, and participation in the production of pornographic material

Learning Disability Nursing at a Glance, First Edition. Edited by Bob Gates, Debra Fearns and Jo Welch. © 2015 John Wiley & Sons, Ltd. Published 2015 by John Wiley & Sons, Ltd.
Companion website: www.ataglanceseries.com/nursing/learningdisability

Recognition of child abuse

Recognition is often dependent on others external to the family. Some children and young people may disclose that they have been abused. In order to assess the child for signs of abuse, the following questions need to considered and answered as part of the history taking:

- Has there been a delay in seeking medical help with a plausible explanation?
- Is the history consistent?
- Can all the injuries be explained?
- Is the child's behaviour and interaction appropriate with the parents/carer?
- Has the child attended A&E or another area of the health service recently?

If the answers to the above questions indicate the possibility of abuse, then a more detailed history, examination and action in accordance with local safeguarding procedures will need to take place. This will involve liaison with social services and possibly the police if there are serious concerns about the safety of the child while a full investigation takes place.

There are certain indicators that raise concerns in the healthcare professional that should be noted. These are:

- Frequent attendance at A&E.
- Bruising or injury in a young baby.
- Unexplained bruising, fracture, head injury in a child who is not yet mobile.
- Parents who present with babies that are not feeding, unsettled or with uncontrollable crying.

A period of observation in hospital may be required to investigate concerns and to support the family. Communication with the General Practitioner. Health Visitor and other professionals is important to ensure on-going support and follow up is provided for the child and family.

Role of the nurse in safeguarding

Nurses who work with children and young people need ongoing education and training in the area of safeguarding to enable them to recognise abuse, and need to maintain excellent documentation in order to articulate their concerns and communications with the child, family and the other professionals involved.

Knowledge of local child protection proceedings is essential as this includes annual level 3 training. The nurse must know who to refer to, who contact for advice, how to make a referral and what documentation needs to be completed, while also continuing to care for the child and family. It is essential then that any anxiety about suspicions and concerns of abuse are made in a prompt manner to the named nurse, named doctor or social worker.

A detailed assessment using the Common Assessment Framework should be undertaken as appropriate. Information sharing is key amongst professionals in safeguarding children.

Legal framework and national guidance for safeguarding children

The current child protection system in based on the Children Act 1989. This Act sets out the law and guidance for the care and the protection of children and young people. The key principle of this Act is that the welfare of the child is paramount. The Court must also ascertain the wishes and feelings of the child under the Children Act 1989 when making any decision that affects them and every effort must be made to protect the child's home and family links.

Harm has been defined in the Children Act 1989 as the ill treatment or the impairment of health or development, including the suffering from seeing or hearing the suffering of another.

The Children Act 1989 also identified the concept of parental responsibility for the child. This includes the duty of the parent to care for their child's physical, emotional and moral development.

Under this Act, Social Care Services have a statutory duty to investigate suspected cases of abuse and neglect. Health Services have a duty to refer concerns and identify cases to social care and cooperate with relevant authorities.

Children in need as defined by this Act are children with a disability, a child who is unlikely to maintain or achieve a reasonable standard of health (or have the opportunity to) without the provision of services by the local authority or a child whose health or development is likely to be significantly impaired without the provision of such services. The local authorities have a statutory duty to provide the services necessary to safeguard and promote the welfare of the child in need.

The Children Act 2004 raised the degree of accountability especially at local authority level, and reinforced the duty of all organisations to safeguard and promote the welfare of children. It provides the legislative framework to support the process of change required following Every Child Matters (2003) to ensure all agencies work together to meet the first five outcomes, which are: be healthy, stay safe, enjoy and achieve, make a positive contribution and achieve economic wellbeing. The main focus of this is early intervention and a shared sense of responsibility by sharing information and integrating front-line services.

Summary
- Nurses have an absolute duty to safeguard and protect children.
- Good documentation is essential.
- Report all concerns and anxieties to Child Protection Teams.

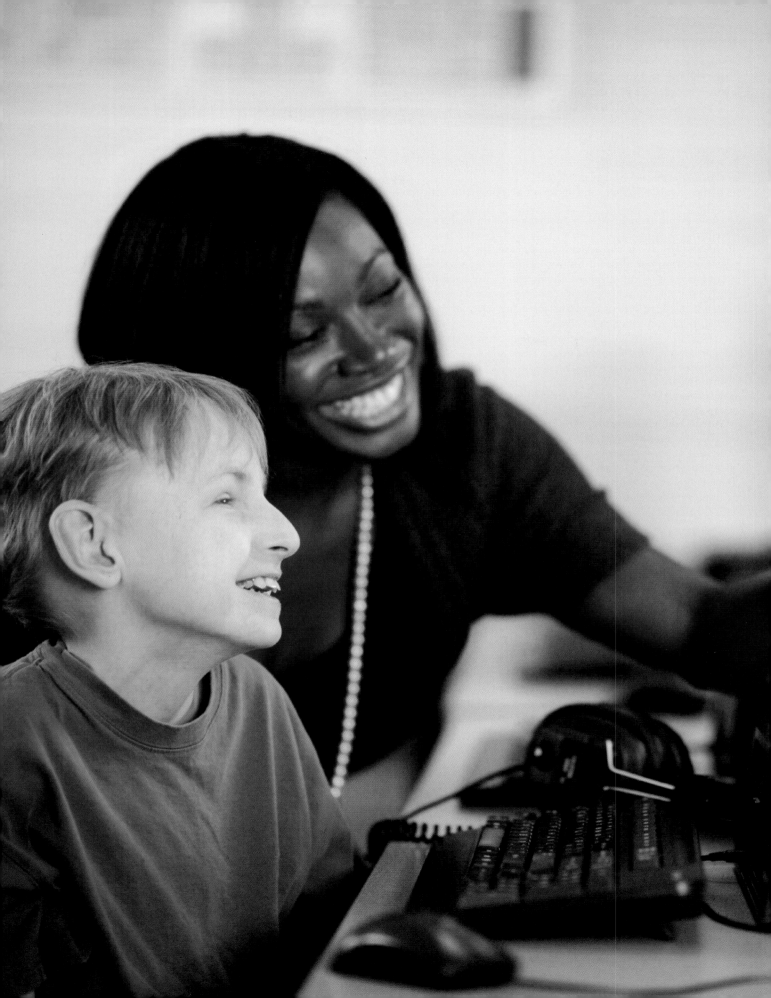

Adolescence

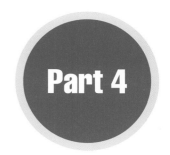

Part 4

Chapters

18 **Puberty** 40
19 **Bullying** 42
20 **Child and adolescent mental health services** 44
21 **Transitions** 46

Don't forget to visit the companion website for this book at www.ataglanceseries.com/nursing/learningdisability to do some practice cases on these topics.

18 Puberty

(a) Puberty poses many questions for the teenager

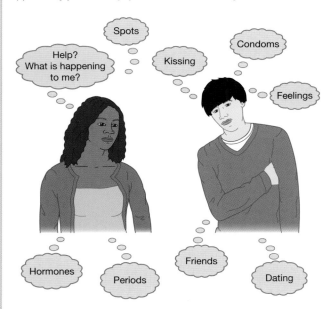

- Spots
- Help? What is happening to me?
- Kissing
- Condoms
- Feelings
- Hormones
- Periods
- Friends
- Dating

(b) There are also many emotions to cope with

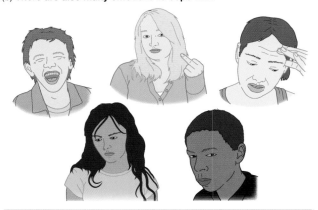

Growing up can make you; happy, sad, on top of the world, down in the dumps, scared, frustrated, nervous, cocky, picky, unsure of yourself, miserable, angry, feel no one understands you.

(c) Working within the Sexual Offences Act 2003

This is important legislation and affects the sex education which may be offered to someone with a mental disorder.

Care workers' offences:

'It is an offence to watch someone else taking part in sexual activity – including looking at images such as videos, photos, or webcams – for the purpose of your own sexual gratification. It is not intended that this should prevent care workers from providing legitimate sex education with an approved care plan'.

This legislation is for adults, however the same provisions should be in place for children, therefore sex education will need to be part of the school curriculum or an approved care plan if being offered outside of the educational establishment

(d) Staff need training too

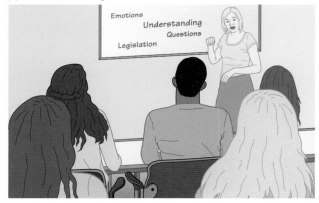

In order for staff to support children with a learning disability going through puberty or coming out of it, they need training

Learning Disability Nursing at a Glance, First Edition. Edited by Bob Gates, Debra Fearns and Jo Welch. © 2015 John Wiley & Sons, Ltd. Published 2015 by John Wiley & Sons, Ltd.
Companion website: www.ataglanceseries.com/nursing/learningdisability

Puberty
Introduction

Puberty is derived from the Latin word 'pubertas', which means grown up or adult. Our bodies are constantly changing throughout our lives. Between the ages of 9 and 15 girls and boys grow taller and bigger and there are physical changes that occur as they grow into young women and men. This takes place over a period of time and gives them time to get used to their adult bodies.

For young people with learning disability (YPwLD) this can sometimes take longer and occur as a delayed milestone. However, when the time is right these changes will take place as the process is dependent on hormones, which are chemicals produced in different parts of the body. These travel from where they are made to other parts of the body which stimulate bodily changes. Hormone comes from the Greek word 'hormon' meaning to set in motion, to start something working. Puberty is a time that is different for each and every child and therefore it is important that a child's physical and emotional development is taken into consideration as a key part of this ever changing time. They will have many questions (see Figure (a) above).

Most schools have a sex education policy that outlines what they are teaching; sometimes parents want to reinforce some of the topics being taught and a good way is for them both to work together so consistent messages are given and understanding is reinforced. This sex education will start to look at the changes happening on the inside and outside and deals with issues such as those outlined in the next sections (these changes do not happen all at once).

Puberty hotspots for young boys and girls

In boys, the hair grows darker and thicker on the face, chest and back, head, arms, legs, hands, feet, shoulders. Chest, penis, scrotum and testicles grow larger. Overall there is an increase in perspiration and oily hair and skin. The voice breaks, testicles start to produce sperm and the penis ejaculates sperm – sometimes during 'wet dreams'. Girls experience menstruation and mood swings, their breasts grow larger, and they will perspire more and get oilier skin and hair.

The role of the learning disability nurse

As children grow up they need to become more independent and are faced with new experiences. They will learn from these experiences better if they are allowed take carefully planned risks; it is quite hard to do this safely without them getting into real difficulties and it can present a real challenge. Adolescents in general, but especially those with learning difficulties, are a vulnerable group and can be open to exploitation and abuse, the lines are fine between overprotection, empowerment and risk-taking behaviour.

Young people often have a lot of questions and it is important that sensitivity is shown when answering them. Remember they are maybe feeling embarrassed and can recognise it if you are too. The nurse wants to create a safe medium for them to be able to learn about what is happening to them and help them to adapt to the changes in a healthy way (Figures (a) and (b) above).

Staff need to be aware of the Sexual Offences Act 2003 and be aware of their limitations when providing any sex education outside of the school curriculum. They also need to have training for themselves in order to empower YPwLD (Figures (c) and (d) above).

Sex education topics are helpful and could include sessions covering hygiene, life stories, emotions, growing and changing, menstruation and wet dreams, body parts, good and bad touching, public/private, different types of relationships, feelings, choices for keeping safe (to include the internet), sex and sexual health, contraception, sexually transmitted infections and access to sexual health agencies.

Summary

• Children/teenagers with learning disabilities may experience puberty as a delayed milestone.
• Sex education is vital and needs to be delivered in an accessible way/format.
• Risk assessment will be a key component when working with vulnerable young people.

(19) Bullying

Types of bullying

Verbal   Physical   Social   Cyber

Specific types of bullying

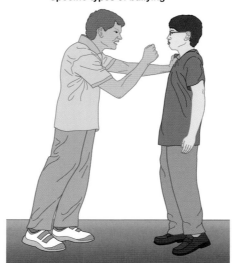

Homophobic bullying
Somebody may bully you if you are of a different sexual orientation to them, for example someone straight might bully you if you are gay and call you 'gay' as an insult.

Sizeist bullying
Someone may bully you because of your size, calling you 'fat' or 'skinny' as an insult.

Racist bullying
People may bully you because of the colour of your skin and call you horrible names linked to your skin colour.

Sexist bullying
People bully you for being the opposite sex, calling you 'weak' if you are a girl for example.

Learning Disability Nursing at a Glance, First Edition. Edited by Bob Gates, Debra Fearns and Jo Welch. © 2015 John Wiley & Sons, Ltd. Published 2015 by John Wiley & Sons, Ltd.
Companion website: www.ataglanceseries.com/nursing/learningdisability

What is bullying?

Bullying can be defined as when one person hurts another person either physically, by hitting or kicking that person, or verbally by calling that person names or teasing the person.

Types of bullying

• *Verbal* – when someone or a group of people is called names, when verbal threats are made. All designed to put fear into someone, to make them feel humiliated or to ensure their silence.
• *Physical* – When someone or a group of people use physical force to frighten another person or another group of people. When someone has items stolen from them and are then forced to remain silent.
• *Social* – Someone is left out of group activities, like games, parties and so on. Designed to make the person feel like an outsider.
• *Cyber* – A new and growing phenomenon. Involves both verbal and social forms of bullying designed to create fear, loneliness and humiliation.

How to identify bullying – the grey area!

In some ways the more extreme the form of bullying the easier it is to identify (for the outside observer at least), but how do you identify the difference between playful banter and bullying behaviour? And is there, in fact, a difference?

For better or worse a significant amount of contact between people is based on 'ribbing', 'mickey taking', 'teasing', or 'banter' the reasons for which are complex and could take up a whole book! Factors that lead to this include the need to put people in their place so as to prevent people from becoming 'too big for their boots'. Another factor to consider is that making fun of the pretensions of people's ways is an attempt by the speaker, the 'mickey taker', to break through the tightly bounded social scripts and roles that people perform that, rather than facilitating intimacy, prevent it, so for instance somebody might make fun of me if I start to use too much 'management speak' or speak too academically, as if 'I've swallowed a book'. This would be a gentle reminder by a friend or colleague that I shouldn't become too fixed in my thinking and get caught up in the ambitions and aspirations of my social class, and can be seen as an appeal to me to remain close and 'more real'.

If, however, this ribbing continued and became more persistent or if it increased in its range of 'digs', or if it continued despite a request for it to stop or was clearly having an impact on the receiver, then it would be safe to say that this behaviour is bullying. The speaker is attempted to humiliate, to undermine the receiver of the comments. S/he is trying to isolate the receiver, trying to perhaps undermine their authority or isolate them.

Learning disability and bullying

Life for a person with learning disabilities unfortunately means facing an element of bullying and is all too often a part of their day-to-day experience. Bullying on a societal level is all too accepted and is threaded into our everyday language. The levels of bullying range from name calling to extreme levels of physical and sexual intimidation.

In a 2012 report entitled Loneliness and Cruelty, Carwyn Gravell interviewed 67 people with learning disabilities living in the community and found that of those 67, 62 had 'experienced some form of harassment, abuse or related crime in the community'. Coupled with this alarmingly high level of abuse was the disturbing reality that, for many of the victims, they viewed it as part of living in the community, with a number of victims viewing the perpetrators as friends: this is so prevalent that it has its own name 'mate crime'.

The experience of bullying on adolescents with learning disabilities

The experience of being an adolescent is suffused with shame as well as the desperate need to be both different and yet fit in. There are huge physical, emotional and sexual changes taking place and there is more often than not a drive towards a more independent life from the family, a time when peers become so much more important than adults.

These enormous changes can be both thrilling and terrifying and as such the risk of feeling overwhelmed is very high. Contemporary Western society is currently obsessed with so called perfection, or as some have called it a 'hyper reality', this aspiration is not real, it is an air brushed reality and therefore can never be achieved, but is constantly strived for. And so these two factors combined can lead to young people with learning disabilities experiencing higher than usual levels of bullying. Why?

Evidence suggests that the changes that are happening to an adolescent are second only to the dramatic changes that occur in an infant, and observations of infants highlight that the emotions attached to these changes are of intense confusion, terror, excitement, anxiety and rage. It is often said that infants are 'thin skinned' and I would argue that this is the case for a significant number of adolescents who are in this huge state of transition.

If there is a desire to fit in, to be the smartest, the toughest, the bravest, the funniest, and so on, then there is likely to be the opposite feelings and fears of being the un-funniest, the most stupid, the ugliest, the weakest. What do young people who are often feeling so much shame about themselves do with this? I would suggest that often they 'bully' those people that are viewed as 'stupid', 'weak', 'ugly' as a way of getting rid of the fears that have about themselves.

Summary

• Bullying can take various forms and is a real problem in all sectors of society.
• People with learning disabilities experience very high levels of harassment and bullying.
• Nurses need to be aware of the pervasive nature of bullying in society and acknowledge it as a problem and support the individual concerned.

20 Child and adolescent mental health services

Signs of psychological distress

Losing interest in activities and tasks that were previously enjoyed

Sexually inappropriate behaviour/disinhibition

Sleep problems

Poor performance at school

Increased anxiety, looking or feeling 'jumpy' or agitated, sometimes including panic attacks

Mood swings that are very extreme or fast and out of character

Feeling tired and lacking energy

Self-harming behaviour, such as cutting, tying ligatures, head banging, ingesting hazardous substances

Isolating self, socialising less; spending too much time in bed

Changes in eating habits and/or appetite: over-eating, bingeing, not eating

Hearing and seeing things that others don't, fixed staring and talking to unseen stimuli

Other differences in perception; for example, mistakenly believing that someone is trying to harm you, is laughing at you, or trying to take over your body

Wanting to go out a lot more, needing very little sleep, feeling highly energetic, creative and sociable, making new friends rapidly, trusting strangers or spending excessively – this may signal becoming 'high'

Child and adolescent mental health Services

Tier 1
Services are usually provided by professionals who are not mental health specialists, such as: GPs, school nurses, health visitors, teachers and social workers. These professionals can refer on to specialist services

Tier 2
Practitioners tend to be specialists who work in primary care settings, e.g. primary mental health workers, psychologists and counsellors based within GP services and schools, etc.

Tier 3
Multidisciplinary team or service working within the community to provide a specialist service for young people with more severe and complex disorders

Tier 4
Specialist services for those with the most serious prognosis. These services include day units, highly specialised outpatient teams and inpatient units, eating disorder units and secure forensic adolescent units. These teams usually serve more than one region

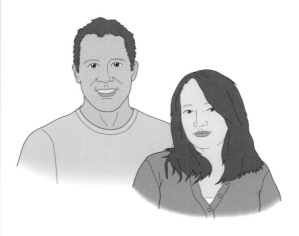

Learning Disability Nursing at a Glance, First Edition. Edited by Bob Gates, Debra Fearns and Jo Welch. © 2015 John Wiley & Sons, Ltd. Published 2015 by John Wiley & Sons, Ltd.
Companion website: www.ataglanceseries.com/nursing/learningdisability

Introduction to psychological distress

Research suggests that psychological distress can manifest from as early as infancy. This can be heavily influenced by factors such as socio-economic status, environmental, biological, culture and socio-political status. This can often present itself in many different variations such as depression, anxiety, confused emotions, rage, psychosis and extreme behavioural disturbances. The key to effective management of such distress is early intervention and effective treatment. There is no time frame on how long such treatment may take. This is something that requires person-centred planning and effective collaboration from all members of the multidisciplinary team throughout. Failure to do so can result in repeated relapses and development of serious and enduring mental illness.

Adolescence comes with its own difficulties and stresses making this an already challenging time of life, add in a period of psychological distress and there is the potential to cause severe disruptions to the young person's development. During adolescence, young people are striving to develop their place within society and this should always be considered sensitively when working with a psychologically distressed adolescent.

Managing psychological distress

In order for adolescents to continue to develop their own sense of identity, CAMH services need to support the young person in their transition into adulthood whilst aiming to reduce the stigma and possible social exclusion that can occur alongside psychological distress. With this in mind, young people should be cared for in the community where possible, treating their mental illness in a sensitive manner with as little disruption as possible. However, there are times where the young person must be admitted to an inpatient setting due to increased risk to themselves or others; if this is necessary then the admitting unit should be specifically orientated to the unique challenges which present during adolescence and the shifting need between self-sufficiency and nurture.

Professionals need to work collaboratively not only with each other but with the young person and their families as well. Adolescents can often be left feeling disempowered by services, which need to be promoting trusting relationships whilst recognising the independence and potential of the young person. With adolescents it is of upmost importance that all those involved in caring for the individual are consistent in their approach so as not to cause further confusion and distress in what is already a challenging time of life.

In dealing with psychological distress, early intervention is key in helping to reduce the stresses and anxieties faced not only by the young person but by their parents and families as well. A detailed background history needs to be taken which should include any family history of mental illness and also all the factors leading to the young person's distress. It is vital that professionals aim to develop strong therapeutic relationships with the young person and their family as communication and talking therapies play a significant role in treating psychological distress. A multidisciplinary approach should be used to ensure that all the young person's needs are being met and this team should strive to communicate with each other regularly to ensure continuity of care.

Therapies available in managing such distress are extensive and varied. These can be provided by a number of skilled professionals, such as psychologists, family therapists, occupational therapists, art therapists and speech and language therapists. These allow the young person to explore and apply therapeutic coping mechanisms that help extinguish those that are seen as maladaptive. This is not to say that the maladaptive coping mechanisms will be ameliorated altogether; however, reinforcing positive ways of coping with such stresses at an early age helps instil confidence that they will be able to manage any future episodes of psychological distress effectively. This also provides an essential platform for the young person to take some form of responsibility in managing their mental health.

Examples of therapies commonly used within CAMH services are Cogitative Behaviour Therapy (CBT) & Dialectical Behaviour Therapy (DBT), both on an individual and group basis. These therapies provide a holistic approach that encompasses many aspects of the young person rather than medication that focuses solely on symptoms. It is important to note that not all therapies are effective and resistance to these can be a common occurrence. Convincing an adolescent that any kind of therapy can be beneficial can prove a difficult task.

In treating young people experiencing psychological distress, medication can be a key element in recovery. It is important to consider the adverse effects of giving medication to adolescents; however, this can be used safely and therapeutically. Many antipsychotic and antidepressant drugs can cause side-effects which are obviously undesirable and need careful consideration when prescribing for young people to ensure the benefits outweigh the negatives. Factors to consider are weight gain, extra pyramidal side-effects (tremor, abnormal face and body movements, restlessness and tardive dyskinesia), sedative effects of many antipsychotic medications, and also the stigma attached to taking these. Those prescribing and dispensing medications need to carefully weigh up the options and should ideally be prescribing medications holistically, in conjunction with other therapies and interventions.

The young person's autonomy should be considered when prescribing medications, they should be given detailed information on the medications they are receiving and what positive and negative effects they can expect. This should be discussed in detail with the young person before prescribing and their opinion and wishes should take priority. The young person should be encouraged to take responsibility for taking their medication where possible in order to promote independence and involvement in their care.

There may be times where the young person does not have capacity to accept treatment due to the level of their psychological distress; in these instances the young person can be given medication with the parents' consent.

21 Transitions

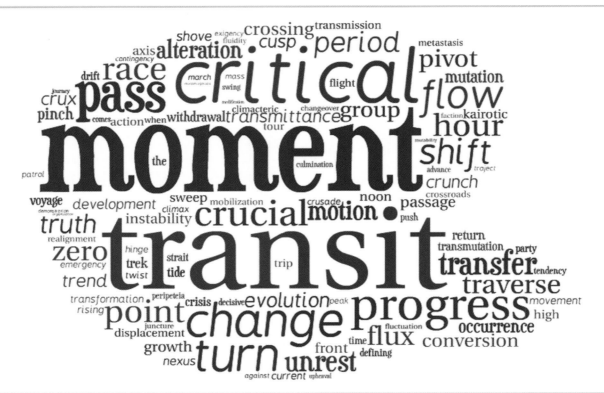

According to the Chambers English Dictionary, a transition is 'a passage from one place to another, state, a stage, style or subject to another'. We all face transitions in our lives, as a child, student, or facing middle or old age. Life is a series of challenges, a series of transitions. How we deal with them, and the support we get, is the key to how well we adapt to them.

The individual

This chapter concentrates on adolescence, roughly 16- to 25-year-olds. This is considered to be one of the most significant phases in the lives of people with learning disabilities. Its importance has been acknowledged nationally and internationally. Transition marks a time where an individual gains greater choice and autonomy as they become independent. There are many internal and external struggles a person goes through in adolescence, such as the challenges of physical and sexual development. There is an increased risk of mental health problems: it could be that they are struggling to hold on to a positive self-image, feeling that everyone is against them, that life is passing them by. Their siblings may have left home to go to university and maybe they are in a sexual relationship and have a job or car. All of these can be out of reach for the individual with a learning disability. This can be painful. The adult world may feel daunting. They may have to face 'a moment of truth', when they have to acknowledge their learning disability. The other option is to deny knowledge of it. This is more problematic. There is an interesting theory, 'three secrets', meaning three aspects of their lives that services and families struggle to discuss: sex, their learning disability and death. The result can be the young person have a lack of knowledge over three important life events. This can increase their potential vulnerability.

Valuing People (DoH, 2001) sets out 11 objectives for how the UK government intends to improve life for people with learning disabilities. The second objective places transition on the agenda. It saw that young disabled people have the right to the same opportunities in education, training or employment as other young people. The challenge here is engaging all the key agencies in the process (education, housing, health, social care and employment) and stimulating multiagency working and commissioning, no mean feat. This can be where the problems begin. The government has put a lot of emphasis on the importance of planning and involving the service user in this.

The family

The family member experiencing transition can be a source of great anxiety. The family may be concerned about how best to manage risk in the future. Many families understandably want to protect the individual. This can result in not letting them take part in life events, for example, not involving them with bereavement rituals or with their sexuality. There are other special challenges for families caring for someone with severe or profound learning disabilities and challenging behaviour. They may have to manage their own mental health, as well as planning for a lifelong commitment. There may be differences in opinion between themselves and professionals; for example, focusing on skills sets while the family are focusing on relationships. This can lead to tensions; services need to work with the family and develop partnerships.

The other key element can be the relationships service users have with peers and staff. In adult services, there are often frequent changes, in particular in staff, with many services having a high turnover. This can have a profound effect on the person with a learning disability. In many incidents, staff can be surprised by their reaction.

There have been a number of studies which show that people with learning disability are vulnerable to the effects of grief or loss. It is important to have an understanding of the grief process. Today's thinking views grief as a psycho-social transition, where practitioners are interested in individual states of mind. This can best be described using the stages model; here the bereaved person would pass through three to five stages starting with shock, denial, sadness, anger, guilt and hopefully acceptance, a useful starting point model for staff.

Part of the nurse's role is explaining the process of grief, one of the reasons they may be vulnerable is lack of knowledge in this area.

The other key educational role for nurses is around sexuality, or otherwise referral to services that can help. It may be important to have more of an advocate role as young people with learning disabilities can receive a poor quality of service, such as the replacement of regular follow-up appointments with as-required appointment systems. They are also more likely to have their health problems either misdiagnosed or overlooked.

For all the above reasons, transition can also be an exciting and challenging time to work with a person with learning disabilities: a period of change.

The nurse can play a part in the individual's development and help service users understand how to access the care and support they might need. Many still need specialist support. There is a lot of planning and coordination involved with a number of agencies at this time. The transition plan can be key. The involvement of the person with learning disability with their plan is crucial to its success. We all need allies, friends, supporters, but particularly people with learning disabilities.

Summary

- LD nurses need to work with young people with learning disabilities in this period of transition, using person-centred approaches.
- Transition has an impact on family and friends, too.

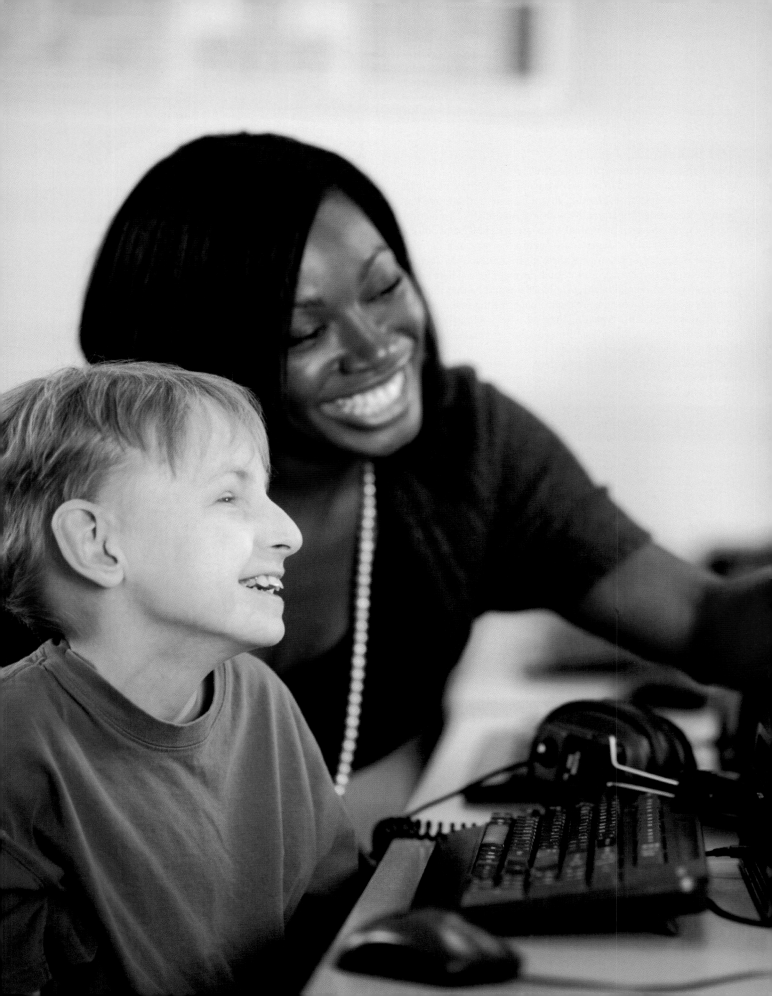

Adults with a learning disability

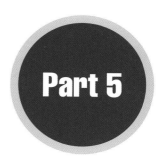

Part 5

Chapters

22 Working with adults with learning disability 50
23 Communicating with people with learning disability 52
24 Sensory impairment 54
25 Living with Autistic Spectrum Conditions 56
26 Epilepsy in adults with learning disability 58
27 Management of epilepsy 60

Don't forget to visit the companion website for this book at www.ataglanceseries.com/nursing/learningdisability to do some practice cases on these topics.

Working with adults with learning disability

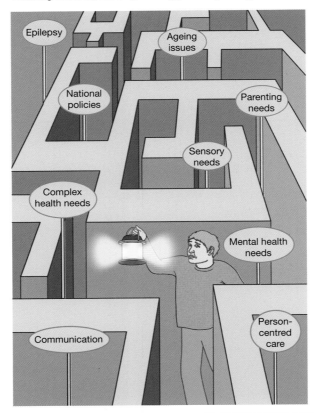

Learning Disability Nursing: Finding your way through the maze

Nurses have to consider the diversity of the varying needs of adults with learning disabilities, including their own approaches to learning disability nursing care.

Nurses' roles are continuing to evolve, from being perceived as doctors' handmaidens to now providing key expertise in nurse led teams, the role of the learning disability nurse is ever changing.

These changes also require the nurse to change their approaches to meet the needs of people with learning disabilities and their families.

With this evolution comes a maze of supporting services along with legislation and policy impacts, with perhaps the greatest emphasis placed on joint working and the coordinated approaches required for the multifaceted requirements of the client group.

Nurses can help steer people through the maze of healthcare and increasingly co-support them through social care.

National policies

Over the last 10 years, key policies have been developed with the aim of improving quality of life and these are based on broad themes:
- citizenship
- empowerment
- having choices and making decisions
- having the same opportunities as other people
- having the same rights as other people
- social inclusion.

Reports such as Six Lives (2009) and the final report of Winterbourne View Hospital (2012) have also shown that widespread service and system failures are evident across a large area of health and social care services.

Educating and supporting services to provide a first-rate service is a role that is further developing for learning disability nurses, for example health liaison teams. This has therefore led to a wider range of support needs for adults with learning disabilities, in which learning disability nurses have had to adapt and develop their own skills in order to meet the diverse needs of the individuals. These include the following.

Person-centred care

Service user-led initiatives continue to be part of the nursing role, and as such the inclusive nature of person-centred planning ensures that individuals are able to have an active voice in their own care. With brokerage within social care now also moving into healthcare, adults with a learning disability will have further inclusivity into their own care packages. Part of that inclusivity is to ensure that people's communication skills are properly understood and detailed within their Health Action Plans and that the people around the person know what they are indicating through their communication (see Chapter 22).

As people are considering their wishes within person-centred plans, supporting people to become parents and enabling families to be together is also an increasing role for nurses. More focus is on providing home-based support rather than centre-based support. This requires the team around the family to ensure that information is user-friendly and the legal aspects made easier to understand.

Complex health needs

The population of children and young people living into adulthood with a range of complex health needs is growing. These needs include a higher incidence of respiratory disease as well as musculoskeletal disorders, sensory impairments and mental illness. As a result people are often presenting with a range of multiple physical, mental and social needs. These needs create major challenges for the person, their families and those who provide services to them. Nurses therefore have to ensure that assessment of someone's needs is paramount in the process of ensuring that these needs are met and multidisciplinary teams are educated in how best to meet the person's needs.

A range of assessments have now been developed such as the PAS-ADD (Psychiatric Assessment Schedules for the Adults with Developmental Disabilities) to ensure that people do not miss out on vital assessments in order to be treated precisely (see Chapter 26).

Many people have some degree of visual and or hearing disability or a combination of both. Some people's sense of taste or smell may also be affected by the drugs they are taking. It is necessary for the learning disability nurse to know as much as possible about a person's vision, hearing and other senses in order to develop the most effective way to approach their learning and communication needs (see Chapter 23).

Damage to the brain can cause learning disabilities. The damaged part of the brain can then become irritable and cause epileptic seizures. Some people might not start having seizures until many years after the damage has occurred.

In some people, epilepsy and learning disabilities can both be part of a syndrome, such as:
- Down's syndrome
- Rett syndrome
- Sturge-Weber syndrome.

Summary
- The role of the learning disability nurse continues to change with the personalisation agenda.
- The NHS needs to acknowledge and fulfil its statutory responsibility to undertake planning that takes into account the workforce needs of the third sector and ensures that the wider NHS workforce is properly prepared to meet the needs of people with learning disabilities and their families.

23 Communicating with people with learning disability

When communicating with someone with a learning disability there are three components you should be aware of:

- Receptive language: Does the person you are communicating with understand what you are communicating?

- Expressive language: How does the person gets communicate with you?

- Social communication: Does the person use body language, conversation, social skills, turn-taking when communicating and do they understand you using these skills?

Aspects to observe when listening

The Communication Chain

Communicating can be seen as a chain process

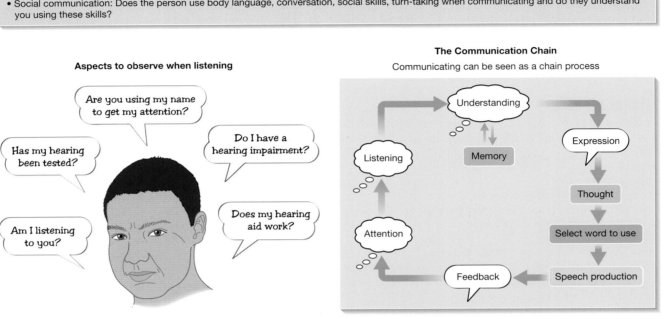

Communicating with an individual with a learning disability means that as a skilled health practitioner we have to be more aware of what we are saying and how we say it. We also will need to be aware of the impact of our body language, facial expression and tone when communicating with people with learning disabilities in order to support that person.

It is essential that the health practitioner listens to the person they are communicating with. By 'listening' we should be aware of not just the things people say but other aspects of communication, as the figure above shows.

Working as a health practitioner for people with learning disabilities should always be done in a person-centred way. You should treat each individual as just that and get to know the person you work with and their preferred communication styles.

Developing a rapport with those you work with and reflecting on the ways the person communicates with other people will develop your skills in all areas of practice.

Receptive language

Symbol use/pictures/photographs (e.g. widget/PECS)

Photos and pictures are a good way to support your speech and help your service user understand you. Before using symbols check your service user understands the level of pictorial support you are using. Photographs are easier to understand than coloured drawings.

Signing (Makaton/Signalong)

Signing gives the service user extra visual information when they are processing what you say to them. If you have a service user with a communication difficulty, then use it! When signing, only sign the key words. Speak and sign at the same time. Use it to support your speech and don't be afraid to use it.

Objects of reference

These are real objects that are used to help the service user understand by giving them the real representation of what you are talking about. This is for service users who find signing, photos and pictures difficult to understand. Objects of reference should be multisensory so that the service user can use all their senses to understand your speech. For example, a piece of towel that smells of chlorine may represent a trip to the swimming pool.

Expressive language

Individuals with a learning disability may communicate through a variety of means. They usually will use more than one of the following to express themselves:
- speech
- electric communication aid
- signing
- communication books with pictures/symbols.
- gesture
- eye contact/eye gaze
- body language
- manipulating/guiding the limbs of carers and other people.

It may take them more time to get their message across than it would take you or I, so remember to give the person plenty of time.

Social communication

Communicating effectively is how people form meaningful social relationships. It is a vital skill in building relationships between service users and the people they come in contact with, as not having the skills for effective communication can lead to social isolation. Many people with a learning disability do not understand unwritten social rules, which most people pick up naturally, such as standing too close to another person.

Remember that a person with a learning disability may have difficulties with:
- interpreting facial expressions
- tone of voice
- jokes and sarcasm
- common phrases and sayings.

Therefore always say what you mean, keep language literal and do not rely on the person you are communicating with to be able to read and understand your non-verbal cues.

Remember:
- Keep language short, simple and clear.
- Check for understanding, if the person walks away, becomes withdrawn, stops making eye contact, becomes agitated or does not respond in the way we would expect them to, it is likely they have not understood you.
- Talk in the present. Time is a difficult concept for many people and yesterday and tomorrow are difficult concepts to understand.
- Give people time to reply. It may take longer for some people to process information, understand what has been said, and express a response.
- Use as many methods as possible to back up speech.

24 Sensory impairment

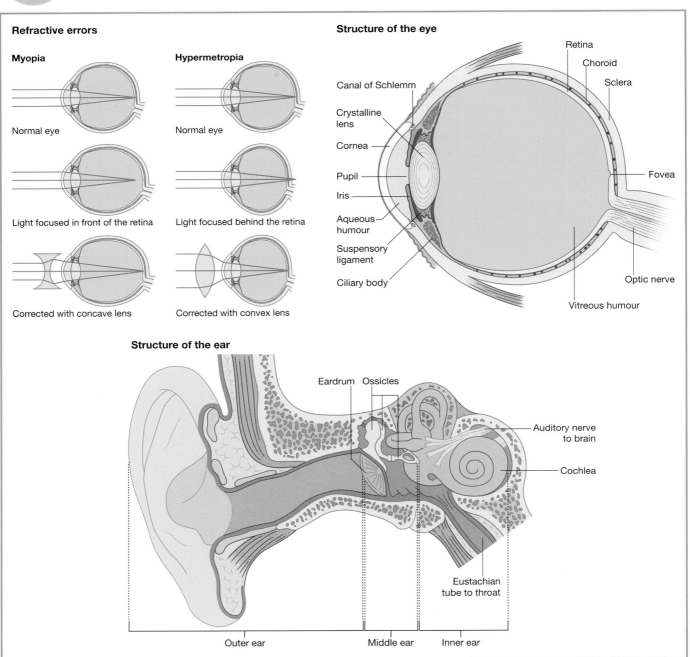

Refractive errors

Myopia

Normal eye

Light focused in front of the retina

Corrected with concave lens

Hypermetropia

Normal eye

Light focused behind the retina

Corrected with convex lens

Structure of the eye

Canal of Schlemm
Crystalline lens
Cornea
Pupil
Iris
Aqueous humour
Suspensory ligament
Ciliary body
Retina
Choroid
Sclera
Fovea
Optic nerve
Vitreous humour

Structure of the ear

Eardrum Ossicles
Auditory nerve to brain
Cochlea
Eustachian tube to throat
Outer ear
Middle ear
Inner ear

Introduction

One in three people with a learning disability will have an additional sensory impairment. Diagnosis of any sight and hearing problem is critical to understanding a person's needs, particularly when they may be unable to communicate any changes in their sight and hearing themselves.

Undiagnosed sensory impairments can be the cause of communication difficulties, significant challenging behaviours and changes in a person's mental health. In people with more severe physical and complex needs the incidence of sight and hearing problems increases significantly. People who have a learning disability should be supported to access sight and hearing assessments to meet their needs on a regular basis, be this through mainstream services or specialist support services.

Sight and hearing problems should be excluded as a physical cause for any changes in a person's behaviour or physical health – an example of this could be when a person experiences sudden and significant sight loss, it is possible for them to experience visual hallucinations. The brain attempts to fill the gaps where the vision used to be. Where the person is unable to communicate their difficulties, it is possible for these hallucinations to be misdiagnosed or interpreted as deterioration in their mental health.

Visual impairments

The most common visual conditions prevalent in people who have a learning disability are refractive errors:
- Short sight (Myopia) – difficulty seeing things in the distance.
- Long sight (Hypermetropia) – difficulty seeing things close up.
- Astigmatism – rugby ball shaped eyeball affecting clarity of vision.

These errors can be corrected with glasses or contact lenses. Individuals with a learning disability should be offered the opportunity to wear glasses to improve their vision. These can be introduced slowly, encouraging their use when the person is engaging in activities that motivate them or when something may be of interest. This is often best introduced on a one-to-one basis to begin with, and the level of input should be on the person's terms and part of their daily routine.

There are other visual conditions which are particularly prevalent in people who have a learning disability. These can be divided into conditions which affect central vision (straight down the middle) and peripheral vision. Conditions which can affect central vision are cataracts and keratoconus. Conditions which can affect peripheral vision are glaucoma and retinitis pigmentosa.

Other conditions which can lead to a reduction in vision are nystagmus (involuntary movement of the eyeball), strabismus (a squinting eye, either convergent or divergent).

It is important to remember that a person with a learning disability can experience a combination of these conditions and therefore have difficulties with both their central and peripheral vision, for example, cataracts and glaucoma. Damage can also be caused to the eyes by other physical health conditions, such as diabetes.

Hearing impairments

Hearing loss can be a result of a congenital difficulty or an acquired loss later in life, and certain conditions or syndromes have a greater prevalence of hearing loss, such as Down's syndrome.

There are two types of hearing loss:
- conductive hearing loss (a loss originating from difficulties in the outer or middle ear);
- sensorineural hearing loss (a loss originating from difficulties in the middle and inner ear);
- and people can experience both these types of loss.

Ear health and ear wax build up cannot be underestimated. People who have learning disabilities experience greater difficulties with wax build up than people within the non-learning disabled population. This can often be through misguided use of cotton buds (pushing more wax into the ear and damaging the skin of the outer ear) or foreign bodies being inserted into the ear. If a person gives the appearance of experiencing a reduction in their hearing, the first step should be supporting them to have an ear examination to exclude wax, foreign bodies or infection as a result of ear poking.

When supporting people who have sensory impairments, it is essential to provide consistent support. If people are supported in a number of different environments – for example, home, day centre, college – the approaches used in their support and care must always be carried out in the same way by all carers, professionals, parents and so on. This applies not only to approaches such as sighted guide techniques, but also to environments, planned activities, and how information is shared and communicated to that individual. It is essential to remember that people who have sight and hearing problems will learn differently as they may not be able to watch or listen and copy others, and will therefore require a structured approach to learn new skills and adapt to new environments.

Summary
- Sight and hearing problems should be excluded as a physical cause for any changes in a person's behaviour or physical health.
- When supporting people who have sensory impairments, it is essential to provide consistent support in all settings and by all professionals, carers, parents and so on.

Living with Autistic Spectrum Conditions

25

Pervasive developmental disorders

Pervasive developmental disorder not otherwise specified (PDD-NOS) which includes atypical autism, and is the most common

Autism

Asperger syndrome

Rett syndrome

Childhood disintegrative disorder (CDD)

Learning Disability Nursing at a Glance, First Edition. Edited by Bob Gates, Debra Fearns and Jo Welch. © 2015 John Wiley & Sons, Ltd. Published 2015 by John Wiley & Sons, Ltd.
Companion website: www.ataglanceseries.com/nursing/learningdisability

Autistic Spectrum Conditions

As indicated in Chapter 15, the number of people being diagnosed with Autistic Spectrum Conditions (ASC) has increased significantly over a relatively short period of time. Thirty years ago autism was considered to be a rare condition and it was uncommon for people to be diagnosed who didn't have a learning disability. In more recent times, as our understanding of ASC has evolved, so has the diagnostic sophistication and general awareness, therefore it is important to note that it is unlikely that the actual numbers of people with ASCs has increased, only the number of recorded diagnosis.

The National Autistic Society (2013) states that there are over half a million people in the UK with autism – that's around 1 in 100 people. Most would agree that around 50% remain undiagnosed. It affects people from all nationalities, cultures, religions and social backgrounds and none are more prevalent than others.

The majority of those diagnosed will have a co-morbidity of a learning disability, this would account for approximately 75% of the overall number, and the further 25% will have autism without a learning disability and would normally have a diagnosis of High Functioning Autism or Asperger's Syndrome. Very often this measurement of IQ and establishment of a learning disability or not will determine the support and services the person with ASC can expect to receive. Historically the vast majority of those with ASCs would be supported for by Learning Disability Services even, it would appear, those without a learning disability. As a consequence of this, the expertise has and remains within the learning disability sector. A learning disability nurse would be qualified and experienced to deal with issues that surround this very different group of individuals. Very often the role of the nurse would include behavioural management support, meeting associated mental health needs, establishing communication aids and ensuring care plans are conducive to the needs of those with ASC.

It is well documented that the group which is causing the most concern within our services presently is those without a learning disability and the remaining 25% of the ASC population. We know that mental health problems for all people with ASC are very highly prevalent and none more so than with this group of high functioning individuals; and they struggle with anxiety and depression amongst other things in a world which can often exclude and isolate them. Unfortunately when these people do need psychiatric help they are experiencing services in which expertise in autism is minimal and the quality of their treatment is questionable.

Sue's short story below helps to exemplify this:

The mental health team seemed to be intent on prescribing medication; "anxiety medication" and "sleeping pills" as well as anti-depressants. I was given a therapist, who I believe was a psychotherapist, although I don't think this was ever specifically mentioned to me, her techniques did more harm than good by causing a huge amount of stress. The only technique she ever seemed to use was to ask me to sit with my eyes closed, listening to the surrounding noise. Although my autism and indeed my hyper-sensitive hearing were not yet diagnosed, the distress this caused me was apparent. When I closed my eyes, my hearing would become more focused. Every little noise, from cars in the street to people talking in the waiting room and even the sound of my mother breathing from the other side of the room, became unbearably loud. These different sounds would build up, mixing together into one blurred noise. Every time I was asked to do this, my leg would start shaking (a sign that I am becoming distressed) and I would frequently start crying. Despite this, the technique would be used every session, despite my mother attempting to intervene. Eventually, I was so upset and distressed about the sensory overload I experienced that I refused to even go in a room with the therapist.

Continually it was obvious that mental health services lacked the understanding of my condition. Because of this, it is easier to reduce anxiety using medication rather than working through it to find techniques that work for each person as an individual. For me, taking medication in itself made my feelings of depression and low self-esteem worse. I found it a struggle to think of the medication as anything other than a failure; I was unable to control my own emotions like a "normal" person.

We often hear the expression that someone is 'somewhere on the spectrum', in clinical terms this expression means very little, however often the term Autistic Spectrum Conditions is aligned with a group of disorders known as Pervasive Developmental Disorders, the figure above shows this group which are often referred to as *the spectrum*. It is imperative that we understand that we are dealing with a wide and varied spectrum of conditions and individuals and although we can make some basic assumptions that those with ASC will nearly always be impaired within the areas of social functioning, communication and flexibility of thought, we can never assume these are going to manifest in the same way.

Summary

- Try to understand which elements of a person with a learning disability's behaviour could be attributed to their ASC diagnosis.
- Additionally, try to understand the elements of their personality or behaviours which could be attributed to their learning disability or mental health diagnosis.
- Whilst there are some 'specialist' autistic services, most people when they require services find themselves within those belonging to the field of Learning Disability or Mental Health.

26 Epilepsy in adults with learning disability

(a) Causes

Symptomatic – a cause is found	Pre-natal, infection *in utero*, labour/birth complication, infection, head injury, brain tumour, stroke, aneurysm, Alzheimer's disease, metabolic disorders, sudden withdrawal of some medications, alcoholism
Cryptogenic – cause is unknown Up to 50% of people diagnosed with epilepsy have an unknown cause	
Idiopathic – cause believed to be genetic Some syndromes linked to learning disability have high prevalence of epilepsy	Angelman syndrome, Rett syndrome, tuberous sclerosis, Fragile X syndrome, Down's syndrome, autism

(b) Classification

Partial seizure Seizure activity that starts in one part of the brain	**Simple**	Person still alert
	Complex	Impaired consciousness and changes in awareness. May be characterised by automatisms such as repeated chewing and plucking at clothing
	With secondary generalisation	Seizures actively spreading from one area to the whole brain
Generalised seizure Seizure activity that involves all of the brain. Loss of consciousness in all types	**Absence**	Briefly staring ahead and blinking
	Myoclonic	Sudden brief jerking movements of arms and upper body
	Tonic	Stiffening of all limbs
	Clonic	Jerking of limbs without period of stiffening
	Atonic	Sudden loss of muscle tone resulting in sudden drop to floor/slump
	Tonic – clonic	Brief stiffening of limbs, then jerking of arms and legs, cyanosis
	Unclassified	An event that describes similar elements to other seizures but is individual to the person

Based on International League against Epilepsy Classification (1981)

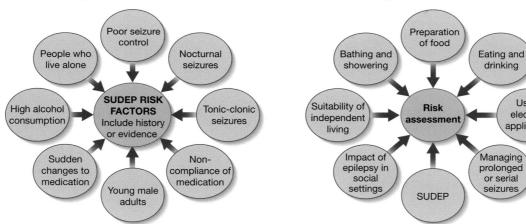

(c) SUDEP risk factors

People who live alone / Poor seizure control / Nocturnal seizures / High alcohol consumption / **SUDEP RISK FACTORS** Include history or evidence / Tonic-clonic seizures / Sudden changes to medication / Young male adults / Non-compliance of medication

(e) Risk assessment

Bathing and showering / Preparation of food / Eating and drinking / Suitability of independent living / **Risk assessment** / Using electrical appliances / Impact of epilepsy in social settings / SUDEP / Managing prolonged or serial seizures

(d) Differential diagnosis

Neurological	Sleep-related	Vascular	Metabolic	Psychological	Other
• Migraine • Tourette's syndrome (motor tics) • Transient ischaemic attacks • Movement disorders	• Apnoea • Night terrors • Sleepwalking • Narcolepsy	• Cardiac arrhythmia	• Low/high blood sugar levels	• Panic/anxiety attack • Hyperventilation • Non-epileptic attack disorder	• Syncope • Alcohol or drugs • Pain • Vertigo • Breath holding • Daydreaming • Behaviours

Learning Disability Nursing at a Glance, First Edition. Edited by Bob Gates, Debra Fearns and Jo Welch. © 2015 John Wiley & Sons, Ltd. Published 2015 by John Wiley & Sons, Ltd.
Companion website: www.ataglanceseries.com/nursing/learningdisability

Definition of epilepsy and clinical presentation

• A neurological disorder characterised by at least two unprovoked seizures due to abnormal electrical activity in the brain.
• Causes disturbances of consciousness, changes in behaviour and emotion, motor function and sensation.

Epidemiology

• Estimated to effect between 362 000 and 415 000 people in England (NICE, 2012).
• Prevalence in UK of 5–10 cases per 1000 population (NICE, 2012).
• At least 20% people with a learning disability across the lifespan have epilepsy, with prevalence increasing according to severity of learning disability (IASSID, 2001).

Status epilepticus and SUDEP (Figure (c) above)

Status epilepticus is a seizure lasting longer than 5 minutes or two or more seizures without a return of consciousness between seizures (NICE, 2012). Convulsive status should be considered a medical emergency and requires urgent intervention with rescue medication such as rectal or buccal midazolam, and/or an ambulance to be called. It is good practice for all people with a learning disability and epilepsy to have an individualised epilepsy care plan and protocol for emergencies.

SUDEP is the sudden and unexpected, unwitnessed, non-drowning death in patients with epilepsy, with or without evidence of seizure and excluding documented status epilepticus. Post mortem does not identify toxicological or anatomical cause of death.

Assessing, supporting and treating adults with epilepsy and a learning disability

Adults with a learning disability can access support for their epilepsy either from their doctor, through neurological hospital departments, epilepsy specialist nurses, or from their local community learning disability teams. It is important that a person-centred approach is taken to both the assessment and the management of the epilepsy, which reflects the four guiding principles set out in Valuing People (2001) and Valuing People Now (2009): rights, independent living, control and inclusion. People with a learning disability should have the opportunity to make informed decisions about their epilepsy management, in partnership with health and social care professionals. Professionals should always follow advice on consent from the Mental Capacity Act 2005.

Assessment

NICE (2012) guidelines advise that a person suspected of having a first seizure should be seen within two weeks of referral by a specialist (a medical practitioner with training and expertise in epilepsy). Furthermore, adults presenting with uncontrolled seizures, diagnostic uncertainty or treatment failure should be seen within four weeks of referral.

An adult with a learning disability may not be able to verbalise details of their epilepsy, could have sensory needs, a shorter attention span and difficulties understanding questions asked, and will need others to support them and also to collate assessment material. This includes:
• History gathering.
• Collecting evidence of seizure description and frequency on monitoring tools or by video (with consideration of consent).
• Ruling out other health conditions which may indicate differential diagnosis (Figure (d) above).
• Risk assessment.

Medical investigations may include full health and blood screening, EEG, neuroimaging, inpatient assessment, video telemetry and ECG. Again, people with learning disabilities will need support to understand and access these. There may be a hospital learning disability nurse that can give support, or support available from the local learning disability team.

Differential diagnosis

Good assessment is vital in order to eliminate any of the causes shown in Figure (d) above, particularly in a person who may have limited communication and ability to describe symptoms.

Risk assessment

NICE (2012) guidelines state that epilepsy risk assessments should include the factors shown in Figure (e) above.

It is important for professionals and carers to recognise that quality of life and independence should be considered when planning management of risk, and that this should be discussed and agreed with the person where possible, or planned under best interest. Aids including epilepsy bed pad alarms, wrist monitors and non-suffocation pillows help maintain safety and independence. Assessment and adaptation of the environment will aid safety and reduce injuries.

Treatment and intervention

Treatment options include antiepileptic medication, surgery, vagus nerve stimulation and a ketogenic diet. Some adjunctive therapies, such as relaxation, yoga and aromatherapy, can also help, but it should be emphasised that these should be used with caution and not as sole therapies.

Many adults with a learning disability will be unable to describe any medication side-effects experienced, and it is important therefore for carers to have appropriate training and to be able to recognise and record unusual symptoms and changes to seizure type, frequency and number. They will then be able to support the person with epilepsy to feed this back to the prescriber. Health education using adapted information helps aid medication compliance for adults with a learning disability, and products available, such as timed tablet boxes, are useful in providing prompts and maintaining independence.

Lifestyle issues

Cole (2010) identified that adults with epilepsy and a learning disability were more likely to experience problems with daily living skills. Epilepsy interrupts consciousness levels, and medication can reduce concentration and impact on levels of alertness. It can be seen that this also impacts on learning and leisure, and people may benefit from further support from an occupational therapist around skill development. Helping people remain engaged in activities that interest them is important, alongside positive, planned risk taking. Activities need to be tailored to appropriate times of day to suit the individual. Someone who experiences seizures first thing in the morning, or is sleepy in the morning, will need activities to be planned for later in the day to fit in with their individual needs.

Physical health conditions and illnesses can cause an increase in seizure activity, and any unusual increase in seizure frequency or duration indicates the need for a physical health check by a medical practitioner to ensure that there is no infection present, or that pain is not a factor.

The impact on self-esteem and social interaction must be considered and positive risk taking discussed to ensure that adults with a learning disability and epilepsy are supported to enjoy a quality of life that encompasses the principles of rights, independent living, control and inclusion.

27 Management of epilepsy

Emergency administration of buccal Midazolam

- Check the person's medication sheet
- Follow the person's epilepsy management plan and time the seizure
- Check the medication; name, expiry date, dosage
- Ensure maximum privacy and minimum fuss
- Try to place person's head in a central position but do not restrict movement
- Place the syringe in the buccal cavity in the mouth (between the gums and the cheek)
- If possible, syringe half the medication into the right side and the remaining into the left (can be administered into one side but separating the dosage helps to prevent seepage)
- Lightly press lips for a few minutes to prevent seepage
- Massage the person's cheek for ultimate absorption
- Make the person comfortable
- Monitor until the person is fully recovered
- Dispose of equipment appropriately
- Ensure information is handed over to the appropriate person
- Record the incident and treatment provided accurately

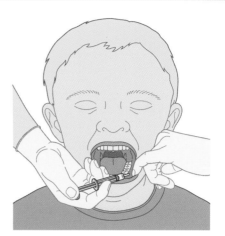

Buccal administration

Emergency administration of rectal Diazepam

- Check the person's medication sheet
- Follow the person's epilepsy management plan and time the seizure
- Check the medication; name, expiry date, dosage
- Ensure maximum privacy and minimum fuss
- Turn the person onto their side if this is possible
- Insert the appropriate length of the nozzle into the anus
- Empty contents completely by squeezing nozzle into the anus
- Withdraw the empty tube whilst continuing to squeeze the tube
- Press the buttocks gently for a few minutes to prevent seepage
- Put the person in the recovery position
- Make the person comfortable
- Monitor until the person is fully recovered
- Dispose of equipment appropriately
- Ensure information is shared appropriately
- Record the incident and treatment provided accurately

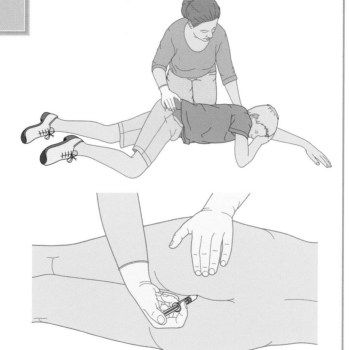

Rectal administration

Learning Disability Nursing at a Glance, First Edition. Edited by Bob Gates, Debra Fearns and Jo Welch. © 2015 John Wiley & Sons, Ltd. Published 2015 by John Wiley & Sons, Ltd.
Companion website: www.ataglanceseries.com/nursing/learningdisability

Epilepsy and learning disability

Epilepsy is seen more common in individuals with a learning disability than in the general population. Indeed, approximately 1 in 4 people with epilepsy will have a learning disability. It also follows that the more severe the learning disability, the more likely that the person will also experience epilepsy. The presentation of seizures in people with learning disabilities may vary and it may be difficult to determine whether an individual is experiencing a seizure or whether it is confused with behaviour. Seizure frequency, duration, complexity and recovery rate can also be greatly affected by the learning disability. Treatment may also be more complex and side-effects of antiepileptic drugs can be more severe.

Whatever the level of learning disability, there are key management strategies to ensure the individual with epilepsy remains safe.

First aid management

- Remain calm and offer reassurance to the person.
- Note the time that the seizure started and time the duration.
- Assess the situation and if necessary remove any objects from around the individual to minimise injury.
- Place a cushion or anything soft under the head to prevent head injury, being careful not to restrict movement.
- Ensure airways are clear by loosening clothing around the neck, chest and abdomen.
- Ensure the privacy and dignity of the individual is preserved – ask those not supporting the individual to leave.
- Refer to Seizure Management Care Plan for emergency treatment guidance or check for ID card or medical bracelet for further information.
- Do NOT restrain the individual or prevent movements – this can cause injury.
- Do NOT put anything in the person's mouth or give them anything to eat or drink until you are sure that they have made a full recovery.
- When the seizure has come to an end, place the individual on their side in the recovery position and maintain observation.
- Examine for and manage any injuries accordingly.
- Record observations at the earliest opportunity and pass this information to carers and appropriate medical professionals.

When to call 999

- If this is the person's first seizure.
- If the person is having difficulties breathing.
- If the person has a seizure which lasts for more than 5 minutes (with no emergency treatment guidance) or if they have more than 1 seizure without regaining consciousness in between.
- If prescribed rescue medication fails to control seizure.
- If the person has sustained a serious injury.
- If **you** feel that the person requires urgent medical attention.

Status epilepticus

When a person has a seizure lasting more than 30 minutes or has a cluster of seizures without regaining consciousness between each one. This medical emergency can lead to brain damage or death.

Emergency treatment

Seizures commonly last for a limited period of time and the individual comes out of the seizure on their own without any further intervention after a few minutes. However, some people may be prescribed emergency treatment for prolonged seizures to prevent the possible damaging effects of status epilepticus. Rectal Diazepam and Buccal Midazolam are both emergency treatments. Both medications come from the Benzodiazepine group of medicines and act on the central nervous system to reduce seizure activity and can be administered by nurses and carers in the community who have received appropriate training. Such rescue medication allows individuals to lead as normal a life as possible and reduces the risk associated with prolonged seizures, whilst reducing hospital admissions and 999 calls.

Rectal Diazepam

Foil wrapped pre-filled rectal tube containing liquid Diazepam administered into the anus. Is usually prescribed to adult in a 10 mg dose but is also available in 2.5 mg, 5 mg and 20 mg doses.

Buccal Midazolam

Liquid formulation available in pre-filled syringe administered via the buccal cavity in the mouth (between the gums and the cheek) or in the nose.

Epilepsy emergency care plan

An individual who experiences prolonged seizures should have a care plan completed by a doctor or nurse. The individual should be involved as much as possible to ensure their informed consent for the treatment. Where the individual lacks capacity to consent, a best interest decision should be made in accordance with the Mental Capacity Act 2005. The care plan should be easy to read and should include the following information:

- Personal/relevant medical information.
- A detailed description of the individual's seizures.
- Any identified triggers for seizures (e.g. menstruation, constipation, lack of sleep etc.).
- Clear instructions including dosage, method of administration and when medication prescribed should be administered.
- Clear indication as to whether a second dosage is prescribed if the first dose fails to stop the seizure and when to seek emergency assistance.
- Side-effects of medication and usual recovery.

The role of the learning disability nurse

Learning disability nurses are ideally placed to liaise with specialist services, individuals and their carers, as part of a multidisciplinary approach to care to ensure effective, safe, consistent and person-centred management of their epilepsy. With their specialist knowledge and skills, learning disability nurses can facilitate and support risk management; care planning, ensure regular review and train carers to empower individuals with epilepsy and a learning disability to live as normal a life as possible.

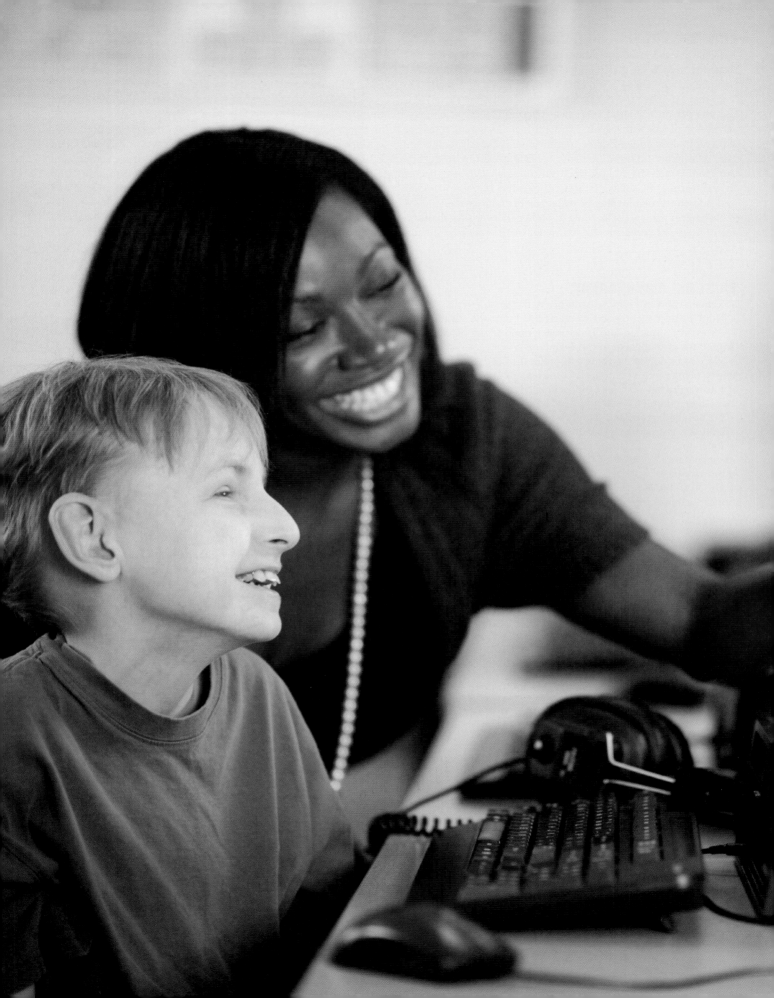

People with a learning disability and additional mental health needs

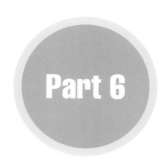

Part 6

Chapters

28 **Managing challenging behaviour** 64
29 **Mental health issues** 66
30 **Personality disorder** 68
31 **Offenders with a learning disability** 70

Don't forget to visit the companion website for this book at www.ataglanceseries.com/nursing/learningdisability to do some practice cases on these topics.

28 **Managing challenging behaviour**

What do we mean by challenging behaviour?

The term CB was coined to denote behaviour that provided a challenge to services and it refers to a variety of different forms of behaviour including:

- Aggression towards other people (kicking, biting, scratching, hitting)
- Destructiveness (breaking furniture and fittings, throwing objects)
- Self-injury (head-banging, self-mutilation)

- Socially undesirable behaviour (such as smearing faeces, regurgitation of food, prolonged screaming, stripping, sexually inappropriate behaviour)

Why do individuals with LD display CB?

CB is often functional and adaptive. It may enable the person to either gain access to things/activities they value or avoid/escape from particular things/events they do not understand or find stressful. What people find stressful is influenced by the following factors:

- Genetic predisposition (e.g. hyperactivity and Fragile X syndrome, self-injury and Lesch-Nyan syndrome, severe overeating and Prader-Willi syndrome)
- Historical factors (e.g. poor parenting, experience of physical or sexual abuse)

- Recent experiences (e.g. being bullied at college or on public transport)
- Current biological state (e.g. feeling tired, hungry or unwell/in pain)
- Current psychological state (e.g. being depressed, feeling lonely)
- Current environment (e.g. noise, temperature, care staff, support and expectations)

Possible consequences of CB

When a person with LD develops/exhibits CB, a range of personal and social circumstances are likely to affect the quality of life of the person and these include:

- being perceived negatively by others
- at risk of suffering physical abuse
- being prescribed medication to manage problematic behaviours
- being subjected to physical restraint and punitive measures

- being excluded from day care, employment, leisure and community settings
- being subjected to material deprivation
- having needs neglected and being avoided or ignored

A detailed assessment of CB in LD is likely to include:

- an accurate description of the behaviour
- an assessment to rule out any underlying physical/ biological factors
- an examination of historical factors relating to the behaviour
- an observation of the person in a number of situations and environments
- an assessment of the person's skills and the carers who provide support
- a summary of the person's strength
- a formulation of the problem behaviour

- an assessment of the environments the person uses and the activities they take part in
- an assessment of the function of the behaviour and analysis of recorded ABC information
- interviews/questionnaires with the person, family members, carers and professionals
- an assessment of the motivators/reinforcers for positive behaviours

Approaches to care and management

- Physical/biological interventions
- Social/environmental intervention

* Behavioural/psychological interventions
* Service models

Overview of positive behavioural support

Environment	Developing skills	Focused support	Reactive strategies
Interventions to address: • activities • outline • noise, light, space etc. • staff skills	• Communication skills • Daily living skills • Coping skills	Interventions directed at reducing challenging behaviour (e.g. reinforcement schedules)	What to do if the behaviour occurs: • listening • redirection • crisis management

Learning Disability Nursing at a Glance, First Edition. Edited by Bob Gates, Debra Fearns and Jo Welch. © 2015 John Wiley & Sons, Ltd. Published 2015 by John Wiley & Sons, Ltd.
Companion website: www.ataglanceseries.com/nursing/learningdisability

Challenging behaviour (CB) in people with learning disabilities (LD) represents a major challenge to service providers and care givers in both community and residential settings. People with LD and CB are known to be excluded from services and often require admission to specialist units for assessment and treatment.

Definition

CB is an umbrella term encapsulating a variety of problematic behaviours which challenge services. The term CB requires further operational definitions to help care staff understand the form, purpose, severity and context in which the behaviour is displayed. The most frequently cited definition of severe CB is: '… culturally abnormal behaviour(s) of such an intensity, frequency or duration that the physical safety of the person or others is likely to be placed in jeopardy, or behaviour that is likely to seriously limit use of, or result in the person being denied access to ordinary community facilities.' (Emerson, 2001)

Prevalence

Determining the prevalence of CB in LD has been a very difficult area and this has led to estimates being made as a rough guide. Variations in the reported prevalence rates of CB in LD are mainly due to different definitions of CB and methodologies employed in data collection. The prevalence trends of CB in LD tend to indicate that:
- CB appears to be more common in large compared to small community settings.
- CB is more common in residential than day services.
- People with LD tend to display more than one type of CB.
- The majority of CB is seen in people with severe LD, but specific CB such as arson, sexual offences and other offending types are seen in people with mild LD.
- CB is most frequently seen between the ages of 15–30 years of age but in some cases may persist into late middle age.

Causes

The literature acknowledges that the identification of possible causes and functions of CB in LD is complex and the causation may involve a combination of the following factors that operate simultaneously:
1 *Biological* – CB is associated with organic brain injury, pre-and post-temporal lobe seizures, autistic spectrum disorders and behavioural phenotype conditions such as Fragile X, Lesch-Nyan and Prader-Willi syndromes.
2 *Behavioural/psychological* – CB is functional, adaptive and consequences maintain behaviour. It is about communication and control, and may be under the influence of external and/or internal events.
3 *Social/environmental* – CB is associated with restrictive/overcrowding living conditions, stigma, discrimination, abuse, lack of support and communication difficulties.

Assessment

A thorough assessment of the possible causes of CB will lead to a good understanding of the reasons underlying the behaviour/s. This process will involve collecting information from various sources about the person's life history, health needs, strengths and abilities, current living circumstances, involvement of services and a detailed functional analysis of the person's purpose and function of problem behaviour. Such an in-depth process will lead to helpful and proactive intervention.

Approaches to care and management

Proactive approaches of responding to CB require the following key principles that should guide intervention strategies:
1 Robust and comprehensive assessment of the causes and functions of behaviour.
2 The nature and intention of intervention should be made explicit from the beginning.
3 Interventions should be subject to risk assessment.
4 Intervention should be evidence based wherever possible.
5 Ensure that the environment support clients' needs rather than challenging behaviour.
6 Help clients to learn more appropriate ways of expressing their needs.
7 Always focus on proactive approaches and avoid reactive and punitive measures.
8 Reward positive behaviour and support clients to overcome skills deficits.
9 Intervention should be based on a trusting and caring therapeutic relationship.
10 Effective multidisciplinary and multiagency style of working.

The care and management of CB in LD may involve a range of therapeutic interventions. Medication is one of the most widely used and popular interventions because it can control a person's behaviour fairly quickly in a crisis situation. Medications such as anti-psychotic and psychotropic drugs are often used to sedate and treat co-morbid psychiatric conditions in LD. The use of medication to manage CB is a contentious issue in LD and there are concerns that too often they are used as an alternative to behavioural support and adequate staffing (DoH, 2001). The evidence to support the use of medication in the management of CB is patchy and inconclusive. Nevertheless, medication may have a role to play but it must be prescribed with caution and is part of an overall treatment plan that includes the above 10 key principles. Behavioural approaches, such as Positive Behaviour Support (PBS), that involve a functional analysis of behaviour can be effective as a means of assessment and management of CB. PBS is a model of assessment and intervention for people with LD and CB that utilises a range of psychological methods and approaches to enhance quality of life and minimise problem behaviour. PBS has evolved by integrating three major intervention strategies that have shaped LD services over the past three decades:
- Applied Behaviour Analysis (LaVigna and Willis, 2005)
- Normalisation/Social role valorisation/Inclusion movement (Nirje, 1970; O'Brien and Tyne, 1981; Wolfensberger, 1972)
- Person-centred values (DoH 2001, 2009)

Summary
- There is some evidence that environmental management such as buildings, structures, fittings, staff (knowledge, skills and attitudes) and service management can contribute to the effective management of CB in LD.
- Additionally, there is also a range of service models across the country (such as intensive support team, behavioural support team and specialist units etc.) that has been evolved to support the complex needs of people with CB and LD.

29 Mental health issues

Stages of assessment

1. Referral for a potential mental disorder
2. Completion of history
3. Meeting with client and immediate carers
4. Physical examination
5. Psychiatric interview
6. In-depth information collected from immediate carers
7. Two weeks' period of data collection including behavioural charting, structured interview and medical investigations
8. Internal staff meeting
9. External meeting with client and immediate carers
10. Presentation of working hypothesis and recommendations

Causes

Biological/physical
Psychological
Social

Vulnerability factors

Brain damage/injury
Low intelligence
Limited communication
Stress
Poor coping skills
Low self-esteem
Risk of abuse
Discrimination
Labelling and stigmatisation
Exploitation
Lack of employment opportunities

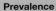

Definition

Mental health is a label which covers different perspectives and concerns, such as the absence of incapacitating symptoms, integration of psychological functioning, effective conduct of personal and social life, feelings of ethical and spiritual wellbeing and so on

Prevalence

People with LD have a higher prevalence of MH compared to general population

Diagnosis

- Beware of the limitations of generic tools like ICD10 and DSM IV
- Avoid diagnostic overshadowing
- Distinguish between challenging behaviour and mental health
- Eliminate physical/biological problems
- Use LD specific tools such as the PAS-ADD and LDCNS to complement generic tools

Common MH conditions in LD

- Mood disorders (depression and bipolar disorder)
- Neurotic and stress-related disorders (generalised anxiety, obsessive-compulsive disorder, phobias and post-traumatic stress disorder)
- Psychotic disorders (schizophrenia)
- Organic disorders (dementia and Alzheimer's disease)

Treatment and management

- Ensure an accurate assessment and diagnosis
- Pharmacological interventions
- Psychological interventions
- Care Programme Approach
- The role of front-line staff/carers/relatives
- Mental health promotion

Learning Disability Nursing at a Glance, First Edition. Edited by Bob Gates, Debra Fearns and Jo Welch. © 2015 John Wiley & Sons, Ltd. Published 2015 by John Wiley & Sons, Ltd.
Companion website: www.ataglanceseries.com/nursing/learningdisability
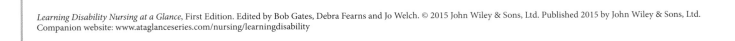

Introduction

The notion that people with learning disabilities (LD) are not susceptible to mental health (MH) issues is an outdated belief and it is widely accepted that this population can and do experience the full range MH problems. The coexistence of LD and MH problems has been acknowledged since the late 1980s and given serious attention in the last two decades due to changes in care practices and attitudes toward people with LD. There is a growing recognition of the MH needs in LD and considerable efforts are being made to develop better MH services for people with LD. However, there are still a number of challenges to overcome particularly around issues of assessment, diagnosis and treatment of MH in LD.

Definition

The Mental Health Act 2007 defines 'mental disorder' as any disorder or disability of the mind.

According to Priest and Gibbs (2004), a mental health problem is said to exist when there is a *significant change* in a person's *mood*, *behaviour* and *thought processes* to such an extent that day to day life, activities and relationships are adversely affected.

Causes/vulnerability factors

It is understood that many people are not born with a MH problem and in many cases MH issues will resolve themselves with or without interventions from MH services. People with LD are exposed to the same risks factors for MH as people from the general population but they have additional physical, psychological and social risks factors that would increase their vulnerability/susceptibility to experience MH problems. Some of the risks factors for MH are:
- Features of learning disability or low intelligence.
- Brain damage and birth injury.
- Limited and poor communication skills.
- Stressful life events such as repeated losses through home moves, frequent change of carers, lack of support, low self-esteem, abuse, exploitation, discrimination, labelling and stigmatisation, failure to be accepted in society and lack of employment opportunities.

Prevalence

There is a wide variation in the reported prevalence rates of MH problems in LD.

There is a general consensus that around 40% of people using LD services have additional mental health needs. There is also evidence to support high rates of psychosis, notably schizophrenia, and high rates of depression and dementia in people with Down's syndrome.

Assessment and diagnosis

Psychiatrists understand, label and treat MH by using one of two key diagnostic tools, namely ICD10 (WHO, 1992) and DSM-V-TR (APA, 2013). These tools are reported to be unsuitable for people with LD mainly because of their over-reliance on verbal communication, which is a major issue in LD. The assessment and diagnosis is further compounded by 'diagnostic overshadowing' where the person with LD is seen as the cause of symptoms rather than assessing the cause of MH in this population, and the difficulties of distinguishing between challenging behaviour and mental illness both of which can present challenges to effective assessment. In light of the above issues, and to prevent under diagnosis of MH in LD, the following tools have been specifically developed for use in LD:
- DC-LD (Diagnostic Criteria for psychiatric disorders in adults with LD – RCP 2001)
- PAS-ADD (Psychiatric Assessment Schedule for Adults with Developmental Disabilities – Moss et al., 1998)
- CANDID (Camberwell Assessment of Needs for Developmental and Intellectual Disabilities – Xenitidis et al., 2000)
- LDCNS (Learning Disabilities version of Cardinal Needs Schedule – Raghavan et al., 2001)

Common mental health conditions in LD

People with LD are known to experience the full range of MH problems and the most common MH conditions include:
- Mood disorders (depression and bipolar disorder)
- Neurotic and stress-related disorders (generalised anxiety, obsessive-compulsive disorder, phobias and post-traumatic stress disorder)
- Psychotic disorders (Schizophrenia)
- Organic disorders (Dementia and Alzheimer's disease).

Treatment and management

The assessment of MH in LD is fraught with difficulties, and without accurate assessment and diagnosis, the selection of appropriate treatment can be very difficult or almost impossible. A range of therapeutic interventions are employed in the management of people with LD and MH problems. These include:
- Pharmacotherapy (antipsychotics, antidepressants, mood-stabilising, anti-epileptics, anxiolytic and hypnotic medications).
- Psychological interventions (behaviour therapy, cognitive behaviour therapy, systemic therapy, person centred therapy and psychodynamic therapy).
- Mental health promotion (intervention to facilitate recovery and meet the needs of users, carers and families).

People with LD and MH problems often navigate between mainstream MH and LD services in their desperate attempts to obtain appropriate MH care. The Care Programme Approach (CPA) provides a framework with identifiable steps to plan and coordinate effective MH care for people with mental illness. Additionally, the role of direct care staff in the assessment, diagnosis and management process is extremely important in avoiding unnecessary and prolonged suffering.

Summary

- Now acknowledged that people with LD may also have additional health needs and that prevalence is higher than in the general population.
- A range of assessment tools and treatments are now available to support people with LD and additional mental health needs.

30 Personality disorder

Definition	PD Clusters	PD Types	DC-LD	Assessment	Management
PD Definition: Personality is disordered, deviating from cultural norms, are pervasive and inflexible and lead to distress or impairment to the individual and/or others			**PD-NOS:** Disharmonious attitudes and behaviours (not cultural norm), not explicable to learning disability, pervasive development disorder, mental illness, drug misuse or physical disorder. Chronic, pervasive and maladaptive across a range of situations. Causes distress to individual and/or others. Impact on occupation and social function		
	Cluster A Odd/Eccentric	**Paranoid PD** (DSM-IV-TR and ICD10)	Excessive sensitivity to rejection, grudges, suspicious, distortion of situations and intent of others, high self-importance, pre-occupation with conspiracy, unjustified suspicion		
		Schizoid PD (DSM-IV-TR)	Not recommended diagnosis for people with a learning disability		
		Schizotypal PD (DSM-IV-TR)	Not recommended diagnosis for people with a learning disability		
	Cluster B Flamboyant/ Dramatic	**Borderline PD** (DSM-IV-TR) **Emotionally unstable PD** (ICD10)	Quarrelsome, conflict with others, impulsivity, lack of consideration of consequences, outbursts of anger or violence, difficulty concentrating without immediate reward, unstable and unpredictable in mood, Emotionally unstable, disturbance of self, involvement in intense unstable relationships, avoidance of abandonment, recurrent self-harm/threats of self-harm, feeling emotionally empty	• Not to be diagnosed before age 21 • Avoid diagnosis in severe and profound ID • Historical factors for developing PD • Physical health assessment • Assessment of skills and abilities • Functional analysis of any behaviour problems • Psychiatric assessment of mental health condition	• Multimodal approach • Pharmaco-therapy (for co-morbid psychiatric diagnosis) • Psychological therapies (CBT, DBT) • Education • Social support • Functional analysis • Risk assessment/ management • CPA
		Histrionic PD (DSM-IV-TR)	Dramatisation, suggestibility, labile, excitement/thrill-seeking behaviours, inappropriately seductive in appearance/ behaviour, fixation on attractiveness		
		Narcissistic PD (DSM-IV-TR)	Not identified in DC-LD		
		Antisocial PD (DSM-IV-TR) **Disocial PD** (ICD10)	Unconcern for others, irresponsibility, disregard for social norms, poor relationships, low tolerance for frustration and aggression, violence, lack of empathy, guiltless, blame others and conflict		
	Cluster C Fearful/Anxious	**Avoidant (anxious) PD** (DSM-IV-TR) **Anxious PD** (ICD10)	Not recommended diagnosis for people with a learning disability		
		Dependent PD (DSM-IV-TR and ICD10)	Not recommended diagnosis for people with a learning disability		
		Anankastic PD (ICD10) **Obsessive-compulsive PD** (DSM-IV-TR)	Doubt, caution, pre-occupation, excessive perfectionism, conscientiousness, rigidity, stubbornness and insistency of completing tasks their way		

Learning Disability Nursing at a Glance, First Edition. Edited by Bob Gates, Debra Fearns and Jo Welch. © 2015 John Wiley & Sons, Ltd. Published 2015 by John Wiley & Sons, Ltd.
Companion website: www.ataglanceseries.com/nursing/learningdisability

Defining personality disorder

Personality refers to the individual qualities of the person that make up their character and influence how they behave across different circumstances. The presence of personality disorder (PD) suggests that for some individuals these qualities are disordered, deviating from cultural norms, are pervasive and inflexible and lead to distress or impairment to the individual or others.

One of the challenges in defining personality as disordered is that personality is developmental. For people with a learning disability there are questions of whether personality develops at the same rate as those of average or higher intelligence. As a result of this the diagnosis of personality disorder for people with learning disability (LD) has sparked debate. Historical views were that it was the individual's cognitive impairment that resulted in abnormalities of personality. More recently it has been recognised that people with a learning disability experience the same life experiences as everyone else and are potentially more exposed to experiences that could be detrimental to personality development. Therefore we must consider the impact of life experiences and other factors on the development of personality.

Prevalence

Total prevalence of personality disorder has been reported as between 6–15% in the general population compared to 1–92% for people with a learning disability. The disparity in prevalence figures for people with a learning disability is due to different methodologies being employed in data collection and this challenges the validity and reliability of diagnosis in this population.

Diagnostic criteria

DSM-V and ICD-10 provide diagnostic criteria for personality disorder. Further guidance from the Royal College of Psychiatrists DC-LD provides advice on applying these criteria to people with a learning disability. The table above provides diagrammatic representation of the classification of the different types of personality disorder, a summary of diagnostic criteria and management strategies for treatment for people with dual diagnosis of learning disability and personality disorder.

Assessment and diagnosis

Currently, there are limited validated tools for assessing PD in people with learning disabilities. As a result, tools used in the general population such as ICD 10, DSM V and Standardised Assessment of Personality have been used and are fraught with difficulties. The DC-LD recommends that PD should not be diagnosed in people with LD under the age of 21 in order to allow for continued growth and development of personality. Additionally, diagnosis should be avoided at all costs for people with severe and profound LD. Due to the developmental debate of personality and cognitive function of people with LD, diagnosis must be based upon a thorough multimodal/multidisciplinary assessment of the following:

- Historical factors for developing PD.
- Physical health assessment.
- Assessment of skills and abilities.
- Functional analysis of any behaviour problems.
- Psychiatric assessment of mental health condition.

A diagnosis of PD in LD is only likely to be possible for a small number of people with adequate cognitive and verbal abilities. Certain subcategories of PD, such as schizoid, dependent and anxious types, are not used in LD because of difficulties in making a differential diagnosis. In many cases, it may only be possible to make a diagnosis of unspecified PD.

Despite diagnosis being contentious it is evident that people with a learning disability are susceptible to developing personality disorders and therefore diagnosis is valid. Diagnosis is also important in ensuring that people with a learning disability are able to access the right support through learning disability and mental health services. Diagnosis must therefore be based upon the benefit to the individual.

Differential diagnosis

The diagnosis of PD in LD is controversial because of its overlap with other psychiatric conditions, autistic spectrum disorders, epilepsy and challenging behaviours. 'Diagnostic overshadowing' may occur when a person with LD is seen as the cause for symptoms rather than examining or assessing the causes of PD per se in this population. The challenge is to carefully assess and differentiate between low intellectual functioning, conditions inherent of LD, behaviour disorders, mental illness and PD. Nevertheless, chronic maladaptive patterns of behaviour which are not fully explained by autisms, limited communication and psychiatric disorders could be explained as due to a personality disorder.

Treatment and management

There is a dearth of research on treatment and management of PD for people with LD. A multimodal approach including pharmacotherapy, psychotherapy, education and social support is recommended. Co-morbid psychiatric illness, substance misuse and offending behaviours are prevalent in people with PD, and their detection and treatment are a priority. Medications are often used to treat co-morbid psychiatric conditions in PD. A range of individual and group psychological therapies have been developed to treat people with PD and LD. These include adapted cognitive behaviour therapy, dialectical behaviour therapy and positive behaviour support strategies. Psychological therapies require the cooperation of the person with PD and motivation to engage in treatment.

Most people with PD and LD have a reduced ability to cope with everyday problems. Help with housing and a range of social matters may be required. Additionally, people with PD and LD are at risk of self-harm, suicide, offending behaviours and other behavioural challenges that can further complicate care management. Implementation of a care programme approach (CPA) is important to ensure risk assessment and risk management needs of the individual are met and health and social care needs are coordinated to avoid potential problems and keep the person on the right treatment pathway. People with PD and LD may have their needs met across a variety of settings, including supported living and residential services as well as specialist treatment centres within mental health and prison settings if detained under the mental health act or criminal justice system.

31 # Offenders with a learning disability

Offenders with ID

Prevalence: Approximately 7–10%. Fairly similar to the general population
Types of offences: Sex offending, arson, property offences, aggressive behaviour and petty crime. Unclear if it is greater than the general population

Risk factors for offending in ID

- Low intelligence
- Sensory deficits
- Increased impulsivity
- Poor social and communication skills
- Social exclusion
- Mental illness
- Personality disorder
- Neurological disorders such as epilepsy
- Autism spectrum disorders and ADHD
- Challenging behaviour and behavioural phenotype syndromes
- Illegal drug and alcohol abuse/misuse

Criminal Justice System

CJS will need to establish whether the accused is criminally responsible with sufficient evidence and if it is in the public interest to prosecute. A 'Capacity Assessment' is undertaken to ascertain as to whether the person:
- Is fit to plead
- Understands the charge against him/her
- Can distinguish between a plea of guilty and not guilty
- Can instruct the solicitor
- Can follow court proceedings

The trial

- People with LD attending court should be supported by health, social and probation services
- Criminal justice liaison team should be able to advise
- If further information is needed then remand to prison or hospital is likely

Disposal

- Fines, conditional discharges
- Probation orders
- Multi-Agency Public Protection Arrangements (MAPPAs). Police and probation to work together in assessing and managing risks posed by sexual or violent offenders
- Imprisonment (health/social services should contact prison)
- Hospital Orders – low, medium, high security hospitals

Admission to hospital under MH legislations

Section 35 Remand for Assessment
Section 36 Remand for Treatment
Section 37 Hospital Order
Section 38 Interim Hospital Order
Section 47 Transfer from Prison
Section 48 Removal to Hospital un-sentenced offenders
With or without additional Ministry of Justice restriction 41 or 49

Treatment and management

- Assessment and management of risk
- Medication
- Psychological treatment
- Multidisciplinary team approach
- Mental Health Review Tribunals
- Courts

Learning Disability Nursing at a Glance, First Edition. Edited by Bob Gates, Debra Fearns and Jo Welch. © 2015 John Wiley & Sons, Ltd. Published 2015 by John Wiley & Sons, Ltd.
Companion website: www.ataglanceseries.com/nursing/learningdisability

Introduction

The term *forensis* is a Latin word for conducting judicial business in ancient Rome. There is not an official definition of forensic learning disability but it is widely understood that it is concerned with the area where psychiatry of learning disability and the criminal justice system (CJS) meet with each other. In practice, the subject matter of forensic learning disability is the clinical assessment, treatment and management of offenders with an learning disability (LD) who may also have a mental disorder. There is a growing interest in the type of services and clinical interventions required to support them.

Learning disability and crime

LD is a heterogeneous group of people ranging from borderline, mild, moderate, severe and profound. People with moderate to profound LD are mostly in supervised care and have little opportunity for serious offending. However, people with borderline and mild LD who live and function independently can be exposed to crime. People with LD who commit crime may be less able to avoid detection compared to the general population. However, there is evidence that the police are less likely to charge a person with LD and/or the crime prosecution service (CPS) may be reluctant to prosecute because of limited chance of securing a conviction. Hence, the labelling of 'LD' may lead to some individuals being excused for their offences and their crimes going unrecorded. Nonetheless, offenders with LD are vulnerable in prisons and there are legal provisions for them to receive appropriate care and treatment instead of a custodial sentence. However, there is a fundamental problem in this area where offenders are not identified as having an 'LD' and they are missing out on the kinds of help and special services needed to support them through the CJS with a view to increase their chances of successful rehabilitation and reduce their chances of reoffending.

Prevalence of offending in LD

The issue of prevalence of offending in LD remains problematic and has long been of concern to those involved in this area. The variation in the reported prevalence rates of offending behaviour in LD is mainly due to different definitions of LD, different methodologies employed in data collection, different locations of studies and changing legislations over time.

Despite the lack of clarity on prevalence figures, it is clear that that there are a large number of people with LD caught up within the CJS. There might be a true association between mild and borderline LD and violent offending. There is some evidence of increased prevalence of arson and sexual offending in LD compared to the general population. Despite the association between criminality and LD, it is difficult to establish whether offending rates in LD are higher than in the general population.

Types of offences committed and risks factors in LD

Offending in LD is more likely to be associated with the consequences of poor socialisation, poor internal controls, lack of social learning, educational underachievement, lack of social skills, poor self-image, mental illness, substance misuse, social exclusion and lack of meaningful occupation. Offences are broadly similar to those offenders without LD but some evidence exists for increased rates of sex offending, arson, property offences and aggressive behaviour. Additionally, offenders with LD are more likely to commit a wider range of offences than those with normal abilities, serious violence is less common and offending is more likely in mild and moderate than in severe. Personality disorder and/or substance misuse together with LD carries higher risks for offending.

Assessment, treatment and management
Assessment

The purpose of assessment is to examine the bio-psychosocial factors that may contribute to the causes and maintenance of offending behaviour. It also investigates for past and present exposure to risk factors for offending and suggests a range of bio-psychosocial interventions to manage future exposure to these risks factors and thus reduced re-offending behaviour. Risk assessment is the process of determining the future likelihood of re-offending and risk management is intended to put in place a range of measures that will prevent re-offending. Research suggests that offenders with LD require a range of services to meet their needs and to manage the risks they present to themselves and to others.

Treatment

Treatment tends to focus mostly on underlying physical and, or, mental issues and long standing patterns of 'challenging' or 'offending' behaviour. Treatment usually includes a combination of assessment and management of risk, medication, psychological treatment, mental health legislations and a multidisciplinary team approach.

Management

The Lord Bradley Report in 2009 demonstrated how imprisoning mentally disordered offenders (MDO) can exacerbate their problems, heighten vulnerability and increase the risk of self-harm and suicide. Home Office Circular 66/90 requires diversion for MDOs, such as cautioning, hospital care and community support, to be considered prior to prosecution. Wherever possible, mentally disordered offenders should receive care and treatment from health and social services rather than the penal system.

Summary

- Offenders with LD are vulnerable in prisons and there are legal provisions for them to receive appropriate care and treatment instead of a custodial sentence, for example through diversion schemes.
- Research suggests that offenders with LD require a range of services to meet their needs and to manage the risks they present to themselves and to others.

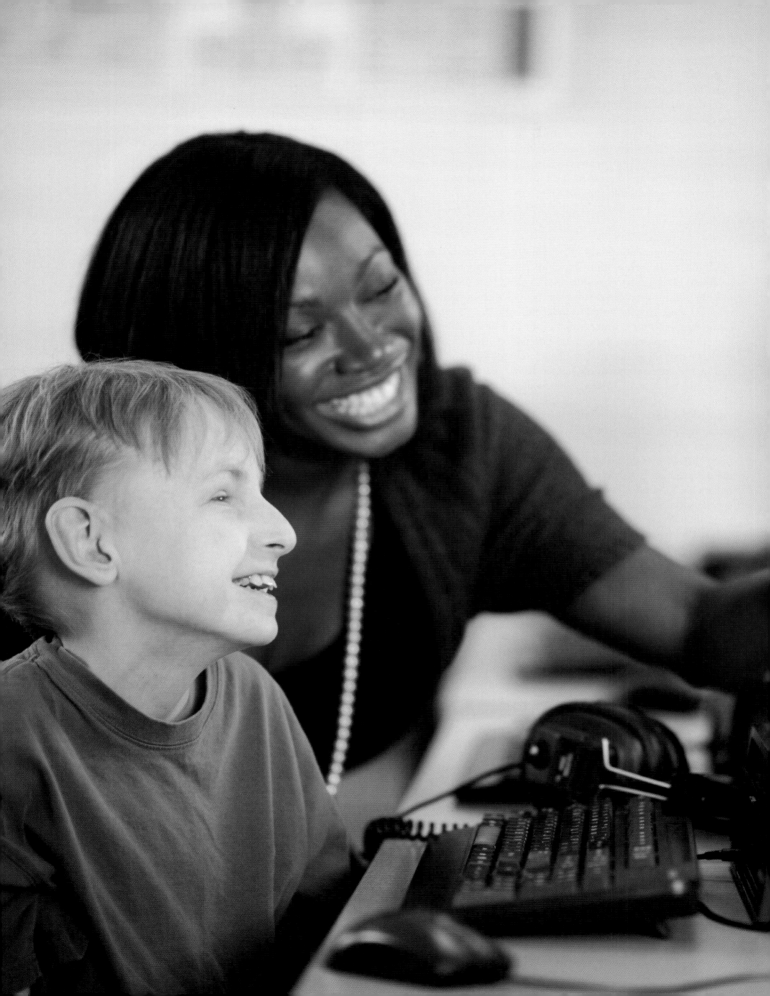

Vulnerable adults with a learning disability

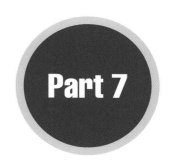

Part 7

Chapters

32 **Mental Capacity Act** 74

33 **Human rights** 76

34 **Equality Act 2010** 78

35 **Mental Health Act** 80

36 **Ethics, rights and responsibilities** 82

 Don't forget to visit the companion website for this book at www.ataglanceseries.com/nursing/learningdisability to do some practice cases on these topics.

32 Mental Capacity Act

(a) The five principles of the Mental Capacity Act

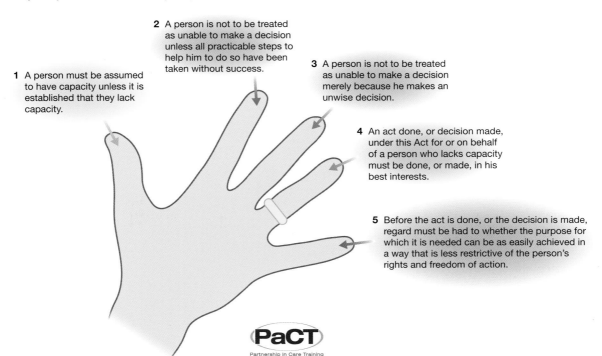

2 A person is not to be treated as unable to make a decision unless all practicable steps to help him to do so have been taken without success.

1 A person must be assumed to have capacity unless it is established that they lack capacity.

3 A person is not to be treated as unable to make a decision merely because he makes an unwise decision.

4 An act done, or decision made, under this Act for or on behalf of a person who lacks capacity must be done, or made, in his best interests.

5 Before the act is done, or the decision is made, regard must be had to whether the purpose for which it is needed can be as easily achieved in a way that is less restrictive of the person's rights and freedom of action.

PaCT
Partnership in Care Training

Source: Reproduced with permission of Hampshire County Council

(b) How do you assess mental capacity?

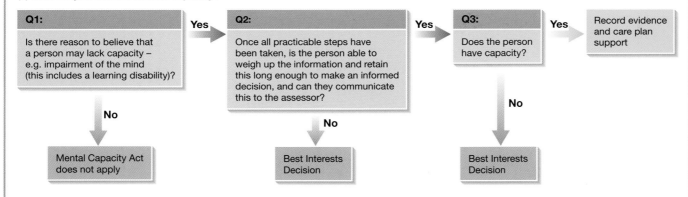

Q1:		Q2:		Q3:		
Is there reason to believe that a person may lack capacity – e.g. impairment of the mind (this includes a learning disability)?	**Yes** →	Once all practicable steps have been taken, is the person able to weigh up the information and retain this long enough to make an informed decision, and can they communicate this to the assessor?	**Yes** →	Does the person have capacity?	**Yes** →	Record evidence and care plan support

Q1 **No** ↓ → Mental Capacity Act does not apply

Q2 **No** ↓ → Best Interests Decision

Q3 **No** ↓ → Best Interests Decision

Best Interests: consider planning meeting to involve all stakeholders including Independent Mental Capacity Advocates (IMCA).

Consider:
- Person's wishes (past and present)
- Person's values and beliefs
- Any advance decisions
- Relevant personal circumstances to consider
- Stakeholders' views
- Benefit versus cost of decision
- What would be the least restrictive option?

The Decision: there can only be one 'decision maker'. In terms of health treatment this will be the consultant undertaking treatment. In terms of other decisions, one person holds collective responsibility, however they would weigh up the beliefs of all stakeholders in the decision.

- Record the decision and evidence
- Care plan support

Learning Disability Nursing at a Glance, First Edition. Edited by Bob Gates, Debra Fearns and Jo Welch. © 2015 John Wiley & Sons, Ltd. Published 2015 by John Wiley & Sons, Ltd.
Companion website: www.ataglanceseries.com/nursing/learningdisability

What is the Mental Capacity Act?

The Mental Capacity Act (MCA) 2005 provides a framework for assessing the capacity of individuals and implementing decisions for those lacking capacity. The act is underpinned by the five principles outlined in Figure (a) above and applies to all persons over the age of 16 and must be followed by anyone working with individuals who may lack capacity.

For the purpose of this Act, a person lacks capacity if in relation to the matter at the material time he is unable to make a decision for himself in relation to the matter because of impairment, or disturbance in the functioning of, the mind or brain (either permanent or temporary) (DoH 2007, p. 42).

How can we help someone to make a decision under the MCA?

In order to assess whether an individual has capacity a process should be undertaken (please refer to Figure (b) above). The individual should be given all of the information they require to make that decision (Principle 2). The following should be considered:

• Communication method: Does the person require an interpreter, use sign or Makaton, picture communication, social stories, real objects or other median?

• What is the relationship with the assessor? Does the person feel at ease with those involved or can other individuals support?

• Can the person learn the required knowledge? Does the decision need to be made now, or can it wait for the person to gain the skills and knowledge, for example a blood test versus emergency blood transfusion?

Capacity is assessed at that moment in time, on the ability to understand and weigh up information. Any assessment undertaken to determine capacity must be decision specific as capacity cannot be generalised (e.g. an individual may have capacity to decide to smoke, but does not have capacity to manage dietary requirements).

Unwise decisions (e.g. a diabetic consuming full sugar fizzy drink) in themselves do not constitute a lack of capacity (Principle 3). It is recognised that supporting individuals when unwise decisions have been made can lead to conflicting feelings (balancing risk management versus empowerment). However it is our duty of care under the MCA to ensure that the patients' right to autonomy is respected.

Some decisions cannot be made under the MCA because they cannot be decided on behalf of another person or another law governs them. These include marriage, divorce, sexual relations, adoption and voting.

Best interests and decision making

Best interests are not defined within the MCA as the decisions and actions covered by the act are too diverse. However, best interests can be considered as the best course of action for the individual, whilst taking into account the previous wishes and preferences of individuals.

The least restrictive intervention must always be considered (Principle 5). This would involve exploring alternative methods that minimise the interference to an individual's basic rights and freedoms. For example, with regard to the diabetic, consideration should be given to alternative options for favoured foods.

Family involvement is fundamental to successfully supporting individuals, including inputting individual's previous wishes or preferences. It is recognised that families may not agree with the decisions proposed for an individual that medical professionals may suggest. Best interest decisions rest with the decision maker, but input from families, IMCA or advocates and carers must be acknowledged (Office of the Public Guardian, 2009).

Where family members may not be involved, an Independent Mental Capacity Advocate (IMCA) may support. IMCA provide independent safeguards for individuals who lack capacity and have no independent body to support their decision making. Further difficulties in implementing the MCA may include where individuals lack capacity and disagree with planned interventions, such as a diabetic who disagrees with necessary diet regime.

Although the MCA does not define time scales for reviewing decisions, these must be reassessed when needs arise, or at regular intervals for ongoing needs. This includes review of previous Mental Capacity Assessments and unwise decisions. Best interest decisions require reviewing, as individuals circumstances may change over time as individuals may develop skills to enhance their decision making process.

What is the role of the learning disability nurse in supporting the MCA?

The learning disabilities nurse possesses a wide range of core skills that include clinical, behavioural and psychological interventions to support decision making and interventions.

Furthermore they can provide vital input to mental capacity assessments and best interest decisions, with key skills including; assessment of capacity for complex patients (Principle 1), providing accessible information (Principle 2), education for individuals, families, carers and other non-learning disabilities professionals (Principle 2), supporting and care planning unwise decisions (Principle 3), ensuring advocacy and person-centred practices (Principles 4 and 5), supporting collection of evidence for decision making (all principles) and ensuring a holistic approach is considered (all principles).

Summary

• The MCA is statutory legalisation, which all professionals and those supporting individuals who may lack capacity must adhere to.

• This aims to both protect and empower individuals who lack capacity to make specific decisions.

• Therefore it is imperative that all individuals supporting people who may lack capacity have relevant knowledge of the MCA; this is something that the learning disabilities nurse can support.

33 Human rights

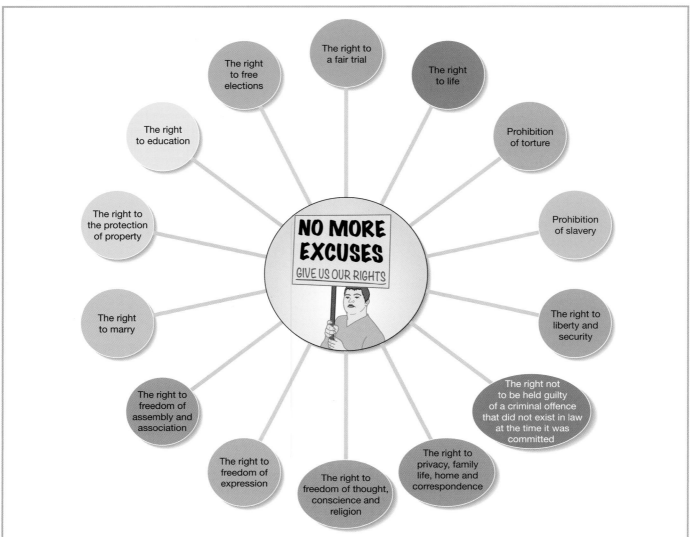

Human Rights Act

The Human Rights Act 1998 came into force in October 2000. The Act makes the European Convention of Human Rights (ECHR) enforceable in the UK. As such the Act did not create new rights but provided new ways for cases to be heard in UK courts, rather than the European Court of Human Rights. The human rights covered under the Act are:

- The right to life.
- Prohibition of torture.
- Prohibition of slavery.
- The right to liberty and security.
- The right to a fair trial.
- The right not to be held guilty of a criminal offence that did not exist in law at the time at which it was committed.
- The right to privacy, family life, home and correspondence.
- The right to freedom of thought, conscience and religion.
- The right to freedom of expression.
- The right to freedom of assembly and association.
- The right to marry.
- The right to the protection of property.
- The right to free elections.

Exercising the rights and freedoms set out above should be without discrimination on any grounds. Not all of these rights are absolute, as some may be conditional and could be denied in certain circumstances. This is partly because a key purpose of the Act is to balance the rights of the individual against the rights of another individual and the greater public good. The Act is not designed to bring actions against private individuals. The purpose of the Act is to affect the way public authorities behave, and to ensure that they attend to the human rights listed above.

It is recognised that adults with LD constitute a group that is vulnerable to having their human rights compromised or denied. The Joint Committee on Human Rights (JCHR) has acknowledged this, and in March 2007 called for evidence to support this assertion. The JCHR commented that:

The extent to which the rights of adults with learning disabilities are currently being respected raises fundamental issues of humanity, dignity, equality, autonomy and respect. It also raises important issues of substantive human rights law such as the right to life, the prohibitions on inhuman/degrading treatment and unjustified discrimination, and the right to respect for family life.

The views of the JCHR reflect that there is an increasing awareness that the human rights of people with LD can be denied. There is an expectation that the Human Rights Act will contribute to a growing 'rights culture' within public services in relation to how people with LD are treated. Valuing People and Valuing People Now (2001, 2009) both supplement the Human Rights Act in supporting a rights culture.

The nurse's role

Working within a person-centred multidisciplinary and multi-agency context in relation to the Human Rights Act, the nurse should:

- Where ever necessary question care practices within organisations if they violate human rights.
- Understand 'whistle blowing' policies and procedures – the NMC Code of Professional Conduct and the right to freedom of expression covered by the Human Rights Act support the right to 'whistle blow'.
- Ensure that you receive appropriate training and support.

Those who are concerned that the human rights of an individual with LD are being breached must:

- take an individual's concerns seriously and seek advice from the CAB or an advocacy group;
- seek advice from a social services care manager or CLDT.
- contact local Social Services Inspection Teams, or Community Health Councils.

European Convention of Human Rights

The ECHR was developed by the Council of Europe in 1950 with the intention of protecting human rights and fundamental freedoms. The Convention established The European Court of Human Rights, which can examine the case of any person who feels that their rights have been violated under the Convention. The ECHR forms the basis of the Human Rights Act 1998 (Human Rights Act b) which made the ECHR enforceable in UK courts. Along with the DDA and other legislation such as Valuing People, the ECHR contributes to the developing 'rights culture' within the field of LD.

Issues of concern

The government has concerns that the rights listed above may be denied to some people with LD. The JCHR has concerns in the following areas:

- *Article 1* – because of fundamental issues associated with humanity, dignity, equality, respect and autonomy.
- *Article 2* – because of the very poor standard of medical care which poses a risk to life.
- *Article 3* – because of the way some people with LD are treated, particularly in healthcare settings.
- *Article 8* – because of a number of factors such as barriers to participating in community activities, which is covered under this article of the convention.

Those working with people with LD must examine their personal practice, and the operation of the services they provide and are located in, and work by using the human rights outlined above as a checklist.

34 Equality Act 2010

The Equality Act 2010 provisions as outlined by the Department for Culture, Media and Sport

The basic framework of protection against direct and indirect discrimination, harassment and victimisation in services and public functions, work, education, associations and transport

Changing the definition of gender reassignment, by removing the requirement for medical supervision

Providing protection for people discriminated against because they are perceived to have, or are associated with someone who has, a protected characteristic

Clearer protection for breastfeeding mothers.
Applying a uniform definition of indirect discrimination to all protected characteristics

Harmonising provisions allowing voluntary positive action

Equality Act 2010

The Equality Act 2010 came into force in October 2010 and replaced the Disability Discrimination Act in England, Wales and Scotland, as well as bringing together a number of other acts, outlined later. The aim of this act is to provide a comprehensive law that will tackle all aspects of discrimination commonly faced by people with disabilities. The act is 'anticipatory', meaning that services, organisations and so on will need to be pro-active and think in advance of the types of adjustments people with a range of impairments may need, rather than being re-active and waiting until an issue arises.

Definition of disability under the Equality Act 2010

A person is disabled if they have a physical or mental impairment that has a 'substantial' and 'long-term' negative effect on their ability to carry out normal daily activities.
- 'substantial' is more than minor or trivial – for example it takes much longer than it usually would to complete a daily task like getting dressed;
- 'long-term' means 12 months or more – for example a breathing condition that develops as a result of a lung infection.

The Act states that a person who has cancer, HIV infection or multiple sclerosis (MS) is a disabled person. This means that the person is protected by the Act effectively from the point of diagnosis.

It also includes people who are certified as blind or partially-sighted.

The Act also covers progressive conditions, defined as a condition that worsens over time. People with progressive conditions can be classed as disabled. This automatically covers cancer, multiple sclerosis and HIV infection from the day of diagnosis.

Aims of Equality Act

To harmonise all the different discrimination laws:
- the Equal Pay Act 1970
- the Sex Discrimination Act 1975
- the Race Relation Act 1976

- the Disability Discrimination Act 1995
- the Employment Equality (Religion or Belief) Regulations 2003
- the Employment Equality (Sexual Orientation) Regulations 2003
- the Employment Equality (Age) Regulations 2006
- the Equality Act 2006, Part 2
- the Equality Act (Sexual Orientation) Regulations 2007

Differences between Disability Discrimination Act (DDA) and Equality Act (EA)

The DDA originally provided protection for disabled people from direct discrimination only in employment and related areas.

The EA protects disabled people against direct discrimination in areas beyond the employment field (such as the supply of goods, facilities and services).

The EA introduces improved protection from discrimination that occurs because of something connected with a person's disability. This form of discrimination can be justified if it can be shown to be a proportionate means of achieving a legitimate aim, for example transgender people can be excluded from specific gender services.

The EA introduces the principle of indirect discrimination for disability. Indirect discrimination occurs when something applies in the same way to everybody but has an effect which particularly disadvantages, for example, disabled people. Indirect discrimination may be justified if it can be shown to be a proportionate means of achieving a legitimate aim

The EA applies one trigger point at which there is a duty to make reasonable adjustments for disabled people. This trigger point is where a disabled person would be at a substantial disadvantage compared to non-disabled people if the adjustment was not made.

The EA extends protection from harassment that is related to disability. Previously, explicit protection only applied in relation to work. The EA applies this protection to areas beyond work.

The EA provides protection from direct disability discrimination and harassment where this is based on a person's association with a disabled person, or on a false perception that the person is disabled

The EA contains a new provision which limits the type of enquiries that a recruiting employer can make about disability and health when recruiting new staff. This provision will help prevent disabled candidates from being unfairly screened out at an early stage of the recruitment process.

The Public Sector Equality Duty

This Duty came into force on 5 April 2011. All public bodies have to consider all individuals when carrying out their day-to-day work – in determining policy, in delivering services and in relation to their own employees. It also requires that public bodies:
- have due regard to the need to eliminate discrimination;
- advance equality of opportunity;
- foster good relations between different people when carrying out their activities.

Specific Duties

The Equality Act 2010 (Specific Duties) Regulations 2011 came into force on 10 September 2011. The specific duties require public bodies to publish applicable, sensible information demonstrating compliance with the Equality Duty, and to set equality objectives. The equality duty covers the following protected characteristics:
- age,
- disability,
- sex,
- gender reassignment,
- pregnancy and maternity,
- race, religion or belief
- sexual orientation.

It also covers marriage or civil partnerships, but only in relation to employment.

Provisions relating to work

- The Act now enables claims to be made for direct gender pay discrimination even where there is no actual comparator.
- Pay secrecy clauses are now unenforceable due to this act.
- Extending protection in private clubs to sex, religion or belief, pregnancy and maternity, and gender reassignment.
- Introducing new powers for employment tribunals to make recommendations which benefit the wider workforce not just the complainant.

Reasonable adjustments

The duty to make reasonable adjustments comprises three requirements. Employers are required to take reasonable steps to:
- Avoid the substantial disadvantage where a provision, criterion or practice applied by or on behalf of the employer puts a disabled person at a substantial disadvantage compared to those who are not disabled.
- Remove or alter a physical feature or provide a reasonable means of avoiding such a feature where it puts a disabled person at a substantial disadvantage compared to those who are not disabled.
- Provide an auxiliary aid (which includes an auxiliary service) where a disabled person would, but for the provision of that auxiliary aid, be put at a substantial disadvantage compared to those who are not disabled.

Age discrimination

The Equality Act 2010 includes provisions that ban age discrimination against adults in the provision of services and public functions.

The ban came into force on 1 October 2012 and it is now unlawful to discriminate on the basis of age unless:
- the practice is covered by an exception from the ban;
- sufficient reason can be shown for the differential treatment, known as ('objective justification').

This ban on age discrimination is intended to make sure that the new law prohibits only harmful treatment that results in genuinely unfair discrimination because of age. It does not outlaw the many instances of different treatment that are justifiable or beneficial, for example, different treatment is permitted by law, such as free bus passes for pensioners.

Summary

- The primary purpose of the EA is to organise the complex and numerous range of Acts and Regulations, which formed the basis of anti-discrimination law in the UK.
- This was, principally, the Equal Pay Act 1970, the Sex Discrimination Act 1975, the Race Relations Act 1976, the Disability Discrimination Act 1995 and three major statutory instruments protecting discrimination in employment on grounds of religion or belief, sexual orientation and age.
- This legislation has the same objectives as the four major EU Equal Treatment Directives, whose provisions it mirrors and implements.
- It necessitates equal treatment in access to employment as well as private and public services, irrespective of the protected characteristics of age, disability, gender reassignment, marriage and civil partnership, race, religion or belief, sex and sexual orientation.

35 Mental Health Act

Commonly used sections

2	Admission for assessment
3	Admission for treatment
4	Admission for assessment in cases of emergency – lasts for a period of 72 hours
5	This is a section used where a patient is already in hospital but not subject to the Act and gives a Dr (5.2) or nurse (5.4) powers to hold the patient for a limited period pending further assessments
7	Application for guardianship – guardianship can be provided by the local social services authority or someone approved by them
17	This section is used to enable patients to have leave of absence from hospital
17a	Community treatment orders
35	This section allows the court to remand defendants to hospital for a report on the defendant's mental condition for a period specified by the courts which should not exceed 12 weeks successively
36	This is used by the courts to remand an accused person to hospital for treatment for a successive period not exceeding 12 weeks
37	Powers of courts to order hospital admission or guardianship. Hospital orders are used as an alternative to punishment and they allow for the detained person to receive treatment for the indicated condition
38	This is an interim hospital order which the courts can impose, for specific periods not exceeding 12 months successively, while making a decision regarding a hospital order – with or without restrictions, prison sentence or other criminal justice disposal
41	Higher courts have the power to restrict discharge from hospital. Section 41 is used in conjunction with section 37 (hospital order) and places certain restrictions
47	This is when the Secretary of State gives transfer directions for a patient to be transferred to a specific hospital. This applies to people with a learning disability
48	Removal to hospital of prisoners who have not been sentenced
49	Restriction on discharge of prisoners removed to hospital – this is as in section 41 and these are called 'restriction directions'
135	With a magistrate's warrant police, accompanied by an approved mental health practitioner or a doctor, can enter premises to search for and remove a person who is believed to have a mental disorder and is not receiving proper care
136	This allows for police to remove people they believe have mental disorder and it will be in the person or the public's interest for them to be taken to a place of safety

Learning Disability Nursing at a Glance, First Edition. Edited by Bob Gates, Debra Fearns and Jo Welch. © 2015 John Wiley & Sons, Ltd. Published 2015 by John Wiley & Sons, Ltd.
Companion website: www.ataglanceseries.com/nursing/learningdisability

Introduction

The Mental Health Act 1983, as amended 2007 (the Act) is a piece of legislation which governs how people with a mental disorder who are viewed as a risk to themselves or to others and could benefit from treatment (however do not voluntarily seek or accept treatment), are provided with assessments and treatment. Assessments or treatment can either be provided in the community or in hospital. There may be occasions when due to the risks presented individuals may have come into contact with the criminal justice system. The Act also makes provisions for how these individuals are disposed of from court or transferred from prison to hospital and vice versa.

The 1983 Act had changes introduced by the introduction of the Mental Health Act 2007. These changes include:
• providing one definition for the term mental disorder;
• introduction of 'appropriate medical treatment' test to avoid detention of people for longer terms unless there is appropriate treatment;
• broadening the group of professionals who could assume the roles traditionally assumed by social workers or psychiatrists;
• giving the patients powers to apply for displacement of nearest relatives and the courts powers to displace a nearest relative considered unsuitable;
• including civil partners among list of relatives considered for nearest relative role;
• introduction of Supervised Community Treatment (SCT);
• new safeguards for patients on Electro-Convulsive therapy;
• reduction of periods when hospital managers can refer patients to the Tribunal if they don't refer themselves;
• provision of independent mental health act advocates (IMHA);
• placing requirement on hospital managers to ensure age appropriate services for people under the age of 18 detained in hospital.

Admission and discharge under the MHA

For individuals to be detained under the Act the following criteria have to be met:

A person can be detained for assessment under section 2 only if both the following criteria apply:
• *the person is suffering from a mental disorder of a nature or degree which warrants their detention in hospital for assessment (or for assessment followed by treatment) for at least a limited period; and*
• *the person ought to be so detained in the interests of their own health or safety or with a view to the protection of others.*

A person can be detained for treatment under section 3 only if all the following criteria apply:
• *the person is suffering from a mental disorder of a nature or degree which makes it appropriate for them to receive medical treatment in hospital;*
• *it is necessary for the health or safety of the person or for the protection of other persons that they should receive such treatment and it cannot be provided unless the patient is detained under this section;*
• *appropriate medical treatment is available.*

The Act defines mental disorder as 'any disorder or disability of the mind'. It is worth noting that the Act excludes drug dependence and alcohol abuse from the definition of mental disorder.

People with learning disabilities and the Act

The Act defines learning disability as a 'state of arrested or incomplete development of mind which includes significant impairment of intelligence and social functioning'. By this virtue individuals with learning disabilities would be eligible for detention under the Act on the basis of their diagnosis, which as defined by the Act is a disability of the mind. Under the Act, however, further provisions have been made to help further clarify conditions when people with learning disabilities meet the criteria for detention. For individuals with learning disabilities to qualify for detention, in addition to the other criteria they would need to be presenting with 'abnormally aggressive or seriously irresponsible conduct' which must be associated with their learning disabilities.

Defining seriously irresponsible behaviour is, however, not qualified within the Act and it is often left to the professionals to qualify what this is. This also means people with learning disabilities can be detained under the Act without any evidence of mental illness as long as their behaviour is deemed to be presenting serious risk to themselves or others.

Safeguards under the Act

There are safeguards put in place for individuals detained under the Act to ensure that their rights continue to be respected. A statutory duty is placed on the hospital managers by the Act to ensure that detained patients or those on SCT have information relevant to how the Act applies to them. The information provided may vary depending on the section the individual is detained under, however it will generally inform the individual of reasons for detention, process for appeal, consent to treatment, provision of IMHAs and information governance. There is an expectation that sections will be renewed and there is recognition that people who are detained may not make voluntary applications to have their sections reviewed. In addition to the reviews done by the Hospital Managers as necessary, patients may also make applications to have their sections reviewed. Where an individual has not made an application for review, the hospital managers can make a referral to the Tribunal for a review. One of the amendments made to the Act in 2007 was the introduction of the Independent Mental Health Advocates (IMHAs) which aim to provide advocates who have a more in depth understanding of the Act to act as advocates for individuals detained under the Act. The nearest relative under the Act also has powers that would assist in safeguarding the rights of the detained individual; this includes the ability to make an application for admission or discharge of the patient from section where applicable.

36 Ethics, rights and responsibilities

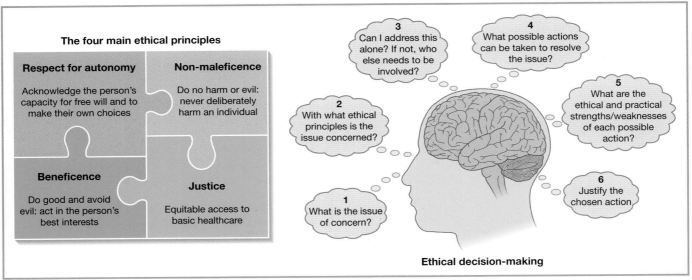

The four main ethical principles

Respect for autonomy

Acknowledge the person's capacity for free will and to make their own choices

Non-maleficence

Do no harm or evil: never deliberately harm an individual

Beneficence

Do good and avoid evil: act in the person's best interests

Justice

Equitable access to basic healthcare

3
Can I address this alone? If not, who else needs to be involved?

4
What possible actions can be taken to resolve the issue?

5
What are the ethical and practical strengths/weaknesses of each possible action?

2
With what ethical principles is the issue concerned?

6
Justify the chosen action

1
What is the issue of concern?

Ethical decision-making

Much research clearly indicates that people who have a learning disability are generally more vulnerable than others in many areas of their lives. This is particularly evident in healthcare, where there is commonly a need for people living with a learning disability to be supported with a variety of decisions, to a greater or lesser extent, in relation to associated health issues which impact on their bio-physical, psychological and social experiences. Healthcare professionals involved in the decision-making process must therefore be both knowledgeable and skilful in analysing the circumstances and needs of those in their care.

But how do healthcare professionals ensure that the support they are providing is actually appropriate and effective? How do they know that the decisions made are the right ones? One of the key roles of healthcare professionals working with people who have learning disabilities is to enable the person to reach decisions about their lives that best meet their needs and upholds their dignity and respect in a caring and compassionate manner. Thus, using a person-centred approach, the decision-making process can be facilitated so that the person with a learning disability can be afforded the rights to grow, develop and experience a healthy, fulfilling life which the person themselves can actively determine within their individual capacity to do so.

In this chapter we will explore how ethical principles can help guide healthcare professionals in their everyday practices in supporting people with learning disabilities. In so doing, the following issues will be considered:
- healthcare ethics
- ethical principles
- rights and responsibilities
- capacity and consent.

What is ethics and why study ethics in healthcare?

Ethics (also often referred to as *moral philosophy*) is a careful systematic inquiry into the nature of morality, that is standards of behaviour underpinned by the concepts of right and wrong actions.

'Ethics is the heart of healthcare.' (Tschudin, 1993)

Everything we do in our direct and indirect care of service-users is based upon a judgement of right or wrong; good or bad. Thus the study of ethics can help us in guiding our professional actions when supporting service users to reach decisions that are in their best interests. Such decisions need to constantly be made using the principles of person-centred approaches where the active involvement of service users, wherever possible, remains pivotal throughout.

Like all of us, people with learning disability will experience a host of life events which may require a variety of decisions to be made, from those that affect ones' everyday routines/activities to the more major events in life, Nevertheless, great or small, decisions have to be reached as to the best course of action. For all involved in healthcare, finding the appropriate course of action must begin with the fundamental and critical question of: '*what decision needs to be made and what decision might be in the person's best interest?*'

The four main ethical principles

- *Principle of respect for autonomy*: to respect an autonomous decision is to acknowledge the person's capacity for self-determination and free will, the person's right to make their own choices and decisions based on their values and belief system

- *Principle of beneficence*: 'do good and avoid evil', that is actions taken must be in the best interest of the person concerned.
- *The principle of non-maleficence*: 'first, do no harm/evil'. *Never* deliberately do harm (either physical or emotional) and always protect from harm
- *The principle of justice*: in the context of healthcare this relates to 'distributive justice', that is, equitable access to basic healthcare.

Capacity, consent, rights and best interests

Any decisions made must be in keeping with professional codes of practice, policy/good practice and legislation.

Consider the above in the context of the decision making process undertaken and ensure you understand, for example, the requirements of:
1 The Human Rights Act 1998
2 The Mental Capacity Act 2005
3 The Mental Health Act 1983 (amended 2007)
4 The Equality Act 2010
5 Department of Health, Valuing People 2001 and Valuing People Now 2009 policy principles:
- rights
- independent living
- control
- inclusion.

Compassion, care and ethical practice

Roach (1992) outlined five components of caring as an ethical endeavour:

Compassion – creating empathy with others by allowing the person to enter into relationships which share joys, sorrows, pain and hurts.

Competence – is one of the first tenets of professional care. Without, 'knowledge, judgement, skill, energy and motivation', there can be no professional accountability.

Confidence – the relationship between patient/client and professional is the cornerstone.

Conscience – is a 'state of moral awareness; a compass directing one's behaviour according to the moral fitness of things'. It often reflects a sense of '*right and wrong*' but in an increasingly complex world, decisions cannot often be simply taken as 'either/or' situations

Commitment – is a quality which keeps a person compassionately by the side of another, or dedicated to a task or idea. It is the human response to a basic belief that caring is, 'the human mode of being'.

Ethical decision making

A simple approach to resolving ethical conflicts or dilemmas:
- State exactly what the ethical conflict/dilemma is that is of concern.
- With what ethical principle(s) is the issue identified concerned?
- Is the issue something that I alone should be addressing; if not who else should be involved?
- What are the possible actions that could be taken to respond to and resolve the issue?
- What are the ethical and practical strengths and limitations of each of the alternatives?
- Justify the specific course of action chosen.

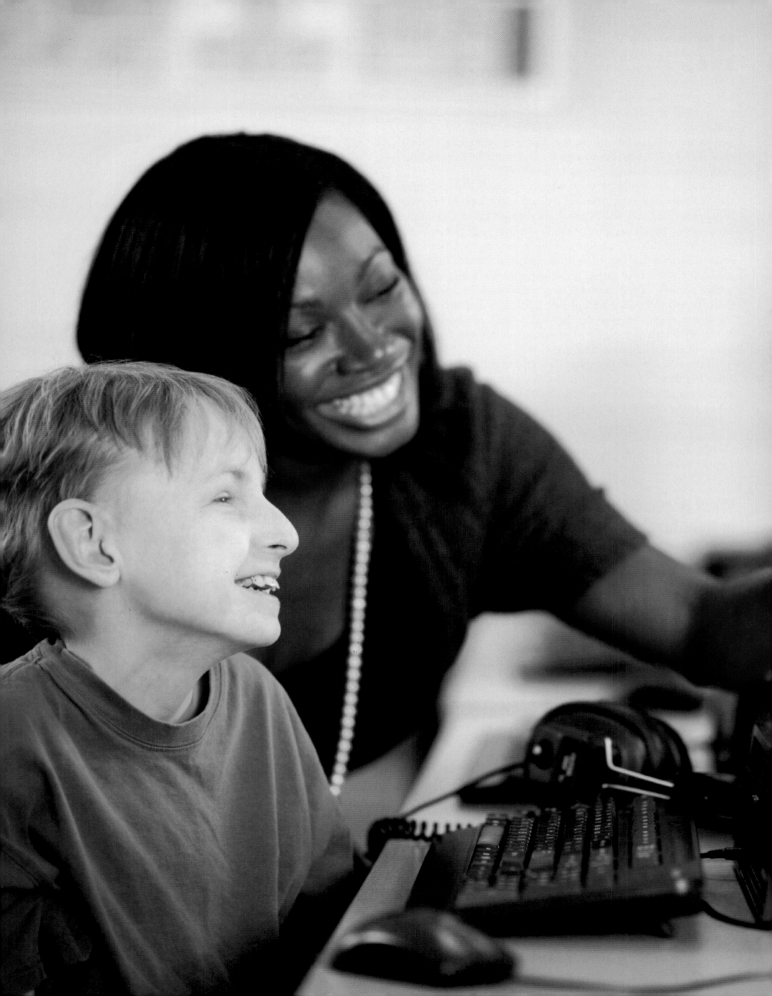

Biophysical aspects of learning disability nursing

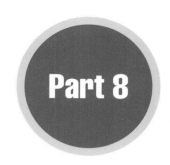

Part 8

Chapters

37 **Biophysical aspects of learning disabilities** 86
38 **Common health issues** 88
39 **The Health Action Plan** 90
40 **Pain assessment and recognition** 92
41 **Palliative and end-of-life care** 94
42 **Dementia in people with Down's syndrome** 96
43 **Sexual health issues** 98
44 **Postural care** 100

Don't forget to visit the companion website for this book at www.ataglanceseries.com/nursing/learningdisability to do some practice cases on these topics.

37 Biophysical aspects of learning disabilities

The information in this chapter highlights the health risks for people with learning disability in order to inform the changes in health behaviour that may be discussed and agreed with people.

Cancer

Cancer in people with learning disabilities (LD) is different than those without an LD.
- 50% level of gastrointestinal cancers (oesophageal, gall bladder, and stomach).
- Reduced levels of lung, prostate, breast and cervical cancers.
- People with Down's syndrome have a greater risk of lymphoblastic leukaemia.

Epilepsy

- 1% of the general population are affected by epilepsy.
- 33% of people with a learning disability are diagnosed with epilepsy.
- 50% of people who have associated complex needs and a severe learning disability (which is of a more complex nature) generally have more than one type of seizure with a complex seizure pattern.
- People may require an increase in care provision.
- There may be continued cognitive impairment.
- People may have a greater need for healthcare input and hospitalisation.
- There will be an impact on lifestyle.
- Greater use of medication will bring the risk of potential side-effects and greater use of rescue medications also has implications for lifestyle and care needs.

Coronary heart disease

- This is the second most prevalent cause of death for people with a learning disability.
- There is an impact from lack of lifestyle choices and associated obesity due to:
  - availability of lifestyle choices
  - inclusivity in activity
- There are risks of hypertension.
- Individuals with Downs's syndrome are at higher risk of congenital heart disease.

Dental/oral hygiene

- Higher levels of untreated disease.
- Tooth decay, loose teeth, gum disease, larger number of extractions.
- Poor dental hygiene and poor diet may have a link with lifestyle choices and:
  - accessible dental services
  - lack of accessible oral health promotion
- Reduced ability to visit to the dentist as behaviour linked to these visits may mean that sedation or anaesthetics are required or not facilitated correctly, sometimes not easily accessible. Often dental problems may take longer to resolve.

- Higher rate of oral complications, including mouth deformities and gum problems in individuals with Down's syndrome.

Diabetes

- More prone to developing diabetes.
- Impacted by the sedentary or inactive lifestyle in people with a learning disability.
- Lack of access to general healthcare.

Gastro-intestinal problems

Helicobacter pylori
- Higher levels in people with a learning disability, mainly when they are living in communal housing or when they are spending time with larger groups of people in workshops or day services.
- Associated with stomach ulcers which untreated can perforate leading to poor consequences.
  - Predisposing factor in cancer of the stomach.

Gastro-oesophageal reflux disease (GORD)

- Affects up to 50% or people with a learning disability.
- Increased in people with complex needs.
- Often associated with specific syndromes, for instance Fragile X syndrome.
- Link to people who may have very different communication methods and a prolonged diagnostic span.
- Link to could also be linked to higher levels of oesophageal cancer in these individuals.

Constipation
- Greater prevalence in people with a learning disability.
- People with complex needs are at greater risk:
  - They may be less mobile.
  - Associated issues with eating and drinking leading to inadequate hydration.
  - Prescribed medication may have this as a side-effect.
  - Over-reliance of laxative medications rather than addressing lifestyle changes.

Coeliac disease
- Greater prevalence in people with Down's syndrome.
  - Gluten free diet, which has implications for lifestyle.

Mental health problems

People who have a learning disability are also vulnerable to mental health problems through a range of bio/psychosocial factors that they are more likely to encounter due to their lifestyle.

Anxiety disorders
- General anxiety.
- Phobias – which may go unnoticed.
- Panic disorders.
- The physical signs of anxiety, such as rapid breathing, muscle tension, and motor agitation, are evident in someone with a learning

Learning Disability Nursing at a Glance, First Edition. Edited by Bob Gates, Debra Fearns and Jo Welch. © 2015 John Wiley & Sons, Ltd. Published 2015 by John Wiley & Sons, Ltd.
Companion website: www.ataglanceseries.com/nursing/learningdisability

disability and could be misinterpreted as some less obvious psychological symptoms might be harder to detect. Anxiety is often seen in those who are on the autistic spectrum who may require more routine and structure.

Depression
- The ability to diagnose may be hindered due to communication difficulties.
- It is easier to diagnose depression in some people with mild learning disability.
- For people with more complex needs and associated communication needs there might be physical signs:
  - weight loss
  - change in sleep pattern
  - social withdrawal.
- Possible atypical indicators, such as behaviour changes that are seen as challenging, for example self-injury, aggression, uncharacteristic incontinence or being unusually noisy.

Schizophrenia
- Three times more likely in someone with a learning disability.
- People could experience a full range of psychotic symptoms associated with schizophrenia.
- Sometimes these may be less marked or less complex.
- Very difficult to diagnose in people with severe learning disabilities since the diagnostic criteria rely on the person being able to communicate their internal experiences.

Obesity
- Levels of obesity in people who have a LD are higher, especially for women.
- Obesity has co-morbidity with other aspects of health and increase the likelihood of heart disease, stroke and Type II diabetes. This prevalence may be dues to lifestyle choices (or lack of choice):
  - Diet choices or pre-packaged food
  - Access to or ability to get to take regular physical exercise
  - Accessible or interactive health promotion material towards a healthier lifestyle
  - The environment may restrict their activity
  - Effects of medication that have weight gain side-effects
- People with specific syndromes such as Down's syndrome and Prader-Willi Syndrome, which are associated with obesity.
- Some people with learning disabilities are at risk of being underweight. This is seen more in people with profound learning disabilities or in those with metabolic disorders such as phenylketonuria.

Sensory impairments
- Sight and hearing problems are common in people with learning disabilities.
- 40% of people with a learning disability have sight problems.
- 40% of people with severe a learning disability have hearing problems.
- People with a learning disability are prone to ear and eye infections.

Sight problems
- Higher prevalence of sight problems requiring adapted assessments to meet their needs.
- Support around the access and importance of eye tests.
- Sight problems may be acquired as people get older, or as a result of brain damage or cerebral visual impairment.
- People with Down's syndrome, cerebral palsy, Fragile X syndrome and congenital rubella syndrome, may have associated sight problems.

Hearing problems
- May never have a hearing test.
- Greater prevalence of ear wax.
- Increased need for a hearing aid.
- Compounded by different communication skills.
- Hearing problems can be are caused by structural abnormalities:
  - abnormal-shaped ear canals
  - neural damage
  - impacted earwax
- People with Down's syndrome, cerebral palsy, Fragile X syndrome and congenital rubella syndrome, may have associated hearing problems.

Swallowing/feeding problems
- People with a learning disability are more prone to problems with swallowing.
- Greater prevalence in those with a profound disability often due to:
  - Neurological problems
  - Structural abnormalities of the mouth and throat.
- Some problems can also associated with rumination, regurgitation or self-induced vomiting.
- Swallowing problems are linked to choking, secondary infections and weight loss.
- Percutaneous Endoscopic Gastrostomy (PEG) is often used to ensure people receive adequate nutrition.
- Often used in combination with oral feeding to enable to the development of swallowing, to eventually withdraw the PEG.
- Advice and adaptions can be sought from occupational therapists.
- Assessments can be undertaken by speech and language therapists.

Thyroid disease – hypothyroidism
- Common in people with Down's syndrome and other people with a learning disability.
- Hypothyroidism might also occur as a side-effect of medications.
- Symptoms can be misinterpreted and include: weight gain/constipation/aching/feeling cold/fluid retention/tiredness/lethargy/mental slowing/depression.
- Untreated this can link to further health issues.

Older people
- Older people with a learning disability have higher rates of:
  - respiratory disorders
  - arthritis
  - hypertension
  - urinary incontinence
  - immobility
  - hearing impairment
  - cerebrovascular disease.
- Also more vulnerable to mental health problems, anxiety and depression, and have an increased risk of dementia.
- People with Down's syndrome are at particular risk of developing early onset Alzheimer's and dementia.
- People with Down's syndrome show changes in brain anatomy associated with Alzheimer's in middle age, although not all will develop the disease.
- Recognition is an issue due to problems around orientation, memory, or loss of skills that may go unnoticed in environments where routine and structure are paramount.
- Down's syndrome is also associated with premature ageing and there are associated additional health needs.

38 Common health issues

People with learning disabilities are twice as likely to experience health problems than the general population

Mental ill health

People with a learning disability are vulnerable to a range of mental health problems; more common are anxiety disorders, depression and schizophrenia

Sensory impairments

More likely to have or develop hearing and visual impairment

Oral health

Poor oral hygiene is common. Almost a third of people with learning disabilities have unhealthy teeth and gums

Obesity

There is an increased risk due to the lack of accessible information, inactive lifestyles which decrease the quality of life and may also lead to the development of diabetes

Epilepsy

Prevalence is 20 times higher in people with a learning disability

Respiratory illness

One of the single most common causes of mortality for people with learning disabilities

Coronary heart disease

This is one of the leading causes of increased mortality for people with learning disabilities. Risk factors include obesity, high blood pressure

Constipation and bowel problems

Common across this population group, although it is more prevalent in people with profound and multiple learning disabilities. There is an increased risk to the population group due to long-term use of medication, polypharmacy and inactive lifestyles

Learning Disability Nursing at a Glance, First Edition. Edited by Bob Gates, Debra Fearns and Jo Welch. © 2015 John Wiley & Sons, Ltd. Published 2015 by John Wiley & Sons, Ltd.
Companion website: www.ataglanceseries.com/nursing/learningdisability

Common health Issues

It is widely recognised that people with a learning disability have a higher prevalence of health problems than the general population. Although there have been great strides forward within the legislation and changing services for people with learning disabilities to ensure a reduction in these inequalities, there is still much to be achieved in this area. People with learning disabilities also experience greater barriers in accessing healthcare.

Overview

• Health needs for people with a learning disability are often unmet and they are at an increased risk of diagnostic overshadowing and developing secondary conditions.
• People with learning disabilities are often isolated, living in the community but not part of the community. Health is often viewed in terms of prevention of a disabling condition with minimum focus on the environment. This misconception leads to an underemphasis on health promotion and on activities that prevent disease and an increase in the occurrence of secondary conditions.
• People with learning disabilities are twice as likely to develop health problems as the general population. This may also increase the number of prescriptions to manage these, thereby increasing the risk of polypharmacy.
• Common health problems include respiratory illness, obesity, coronary heart disease and bowel and bladder difficulties, among others.
• People with learning disabilities are also at an increased risk of developing mental health problems than the general population.
• With increased longevity and improved social circumstances, people with a learning disability remain at increased risk of early death in comparison with the general population.
• People with learning disabilities are less likely to be offered preventative healthcare such as screening for, for example, breast cancers, blood pressures, diabetes.
• People with a learning disability may sometimes find it difficult to explain their symptoms or to explain when they feel unwell; therefore regular health checks are important in reducing these health inequalities.
• People with learning disability may also experience communication difficulties in understanding their symptoms and reporting their health concerns or symptoms to healthcare professionals.

Common health issues

Respiratory illness/conditions

Respiratory illness is possibly the leading cause of death for people with a learning disability. It is reported that the mortality rates are at least twice as high when compared to that of the general population. Respiratory illness is more prevalent in people with multiple and profound learning disabilities who are immobile and for people who are obese. Some of the reasons for this include difficulties with swallowing, poor cough reflex, immobility and difficulties with positioning.

Obesity

People with learning disabilities are at high risk of becoming obese and this is a major health concern. In particular, people with mild learning disabilities, living in the community, are reported to have a relatively high calorie intake. Other factors such as inactive lifestyles and low levels of physical activity are also major contributory

factors. Lower physical exertion and obesity appear to be the most prominent modifiable risk factors to reduce the risk of cardiovascular disease.

Epilepsy

Epilepsy is a prevalent condition experienced by people with a learning disability. It is often associated with people with multiple and profound learning disabilities. The prevalence of epilepsy for people with learning disabilities is twenty times higher than the general population.

Coronary heart disease

This is one of the most common causes of death for people with a learning disability. In particular people with Down's syndrome are at an increased risk for mitral valve prolapse and valvular regurgitation. The incidence rates are expected to increase with time due to a longer life expectancy and changes in lifestyles. People with learning disabilities are more likely to develop hypertension and obesity, and lack exercise, all of which are contributory risk factors for ischaemic heart disease.

Constipation

Chronic constipation is frequently common in people with a learning disability. Communication difficulties and diagnostic overshadowing may result in this being missed by clinicians. Chronic constipation is more prevalent in people with profound learning disabilities who are less mobile. Contributory factors include the long term use of some medications and an inactive lifestyle with little or no exercise and limited food choice.

Cancer

People with learning disabilities are at increased risk of developing cancers of the gastro-intestinal tract, such as oesophageal, stomach and pancreatic cancer. There is also a high prevalence of *helicobacter pylori*, which is linked to stomach cancer.

Mental health

People with learning disabilities are vulnerable to a range of psychiatric disorders, the most common of which are depression, anxiety disorders, schizophrenia and dementia. Children and young adults with learning disabilities are possibly four times as likely to experience mental health problems as their peers without learning disabilities.

Depression and anxiety disorders

People with learning disabilities experience the full range of affective disorders experienced by the rest of the population. Often people with a learning disability may not be able to express verbally how they are feeling and their actions may give some indication of depression. Autism and other developmental disorders may increase the susceptibility of anxiety disorders. Contributory factors may include inadequate social support, poor coping skills or the lack of social and cognitive resources to cope.

Schizophrenia

There is some evidence to indicate that people with a learning disability are three times more likely to experience schizophrenia than the general population. Prevalence rates appear to be higher for adults with learning disabilities from ethnic minority groups.

39 The Health Action Plan

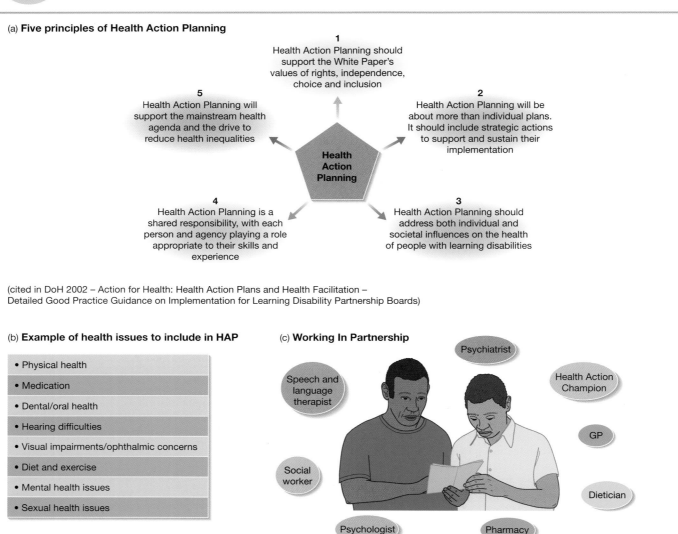

(a) Five principles of Health Action Planning

1
Health Action Planning should support the White Paper's values of rights, independence, choice and inclusion

5
Health Action Planning will support the mainstream health agenda and the drive to reduce health inequalities

2
Health Action Planning will be about more than individual plans. It should include strategic actions to support and sustain their implementation

Health Action Planning

4
Health Action Planning is a shared responsibility, with each person and agency playing a role appropriate to their skills and experience

3
Health Action Planning should address both individual and societal influences on the health of people with learning disabilities

(cited in DoH 2002 – Action for Health: Health Action Plans and Health Facilitation – Detailed Good Practice Guidance on Implementation for Learning Disability Partnership Boards)

(b) Example of health issues to include in HAP

- Physical health
- Medication
- Dental/oral health
- Hearing difficulties
- Visual impairments/ophthalmic concerns
- Diet and exercise
- Mental health issues
- Sexual health issues

(c) Working In Partnership

Psychiatrist

Speech and language therapist

Health Action Champion

Social worker

GP

Dietician

Psychologist

Pharmacy

Learning Disability Nursing at a Glance, First Edition. Edited by Bob Gates, Debra Fearns and Jo Welch. © 2015 John Wiley & Sons, Ltd. Published 2015 by John Wiley & Sons, Ltd.
Companion website: www.ataglanceseries.com/nursing/learningdisability

Definition

A Health Action Plan (HAP) is a document pertaining to a learning disabled person's health. It is written between the person with learning disabilities and the appropriate healthcare professional who is going to support their health needs. The process can be facilitated by a learning disability nurse in conjunction with the individual and the relevant healthcare professional who is going to be responsible for the delivery of the service and/or procedure.

What is a Health Action Plan?

Health Action Plans were introduced in the Valuing People 2001 White Paper, to redress the inequalities in health care provision experienced by people with a learning disability. HAPs can be viewed as a tool to ensure that a person with a learning disability is provided with an appropriate level of support and guidance when accessing healthcare services, thus ensuring and maintaining improvement in standards of healthcare provision for the learning disabled community. A key function of a HAP is to enable the person with learning disabilities to understand the relevance of a healthy diet and lifestyle. Also, it can be used as an educational tool in health promotion and maintenance of good health. In addition, a HAP can identify areas of the health which may necessitate additional monitoring.

Why do we need a Health Action Plan for people with a learning disability?

Prior to the closure of institutions, the healthcare needs of the person with learning disabilities were met by the organisation in which they resided. With the closure of the institutions and the emphasis on community living, it became a requirement for the GP services to provide healthcare for the learning disabled population. However, community integration and adequate healthcare provision for some was, and continues to be, a difficult process, fraught with prejudices, discrimination and inequalities. Valuing People: A New Strategy for Learning Disability for the 21st Century has at its core the principles of rights, independence, choice and inclusion, which are contained in legislation that confers rights and equality to all citizens. This includes the right to healthcare and equality in its provision. The publication of MENCAP's Death by Indifference Report 2007, served as a turning point in healthcare provision for people with learning disabilities accessing and utilising mainstream acute health facilities and services. Further reports such as Health Care for All 2008, Valuing People Now 2009 and No Health Without Mental Health 2011, together with various voluntary sector and support groups, highlight how attempts are being made to improve healthcare provision for people with LD (see Figure (a) above).

Contents of a Health Action Plan

As there is no set design for what a HAP should look like, it is very much up to the service user and their health professional to determine its layout and how it best meets the needs of the learning disabled person.

A HAP contains areas of health concerns for the individual, which are accompanied with an action plan for each concern identifying who is going to do what and when and how it is going to be facilitated. It may also contain the local Health Access Champion's details (see Figure (b) above).

Monitoring and evaluation

The monitoring and review of health issues is an essential component of the health action process. So, when developing a HAP, progress, review and evaluation dates will need to be identified with the appropriate professional or clinician. When reviewing the individual's health issues the reviewer should establish that the necessary level of support was provided in order to achieve the identified actions. Also, the effectiveness of the action and intervention will need evaluating together with the identification of any future action.

The role of the learning disabilities nurse in Health Action Planning

The learning disability nurse has a pivotal role in the development and facilitating the implementation of the HAP. Apart from using their skills to develop a therapeutic relationship with the individual, they are able to provide the necessary one-to-one support to assist the person with learning disabilities to access healthcare services. While it is essential that access to services is obtained, it is even more vital that the recipient is able to understand the information provided, so they are able to make an informed decision regarding their health and proposed treatment and/or service being offered. Otherwise it could be concluded that lip service is being paid to the person with learning disability's rights, dignity and choice. To ensure that such lip service does not become common practice, the learning disability nurse is required to use both their nursing knowledge and skills, while working in partnership with the individual, to translate the often jargonised information and procedure into a more usable and understandable format which meets the learning disabled person's needs.

As a care coordinator, the nurse not only assists in the development of HAPs, they also ensure that such plans are implemented. In taking government documentation and legislation and translating it into practice, the nurse ensures that the person with learning disabilities, mainstream services and clinicians receive the required level of support to ensure safe and effective delivery of care and services. Forging links and breaking down barriers between services ensures that reasonable adjustments within mainstream services and professionals becomes a reality, influencing the development of future services. This in turn leads to greater empowerment of the person with learning disabilities and potentially greater health outcomes.

Pain assessment and recognition

Family/carers pain indicator review example

Pain Picture - Known indicators of pain for...

Indicator	Family Observation Normal	Family Observation Pain
Skin colour	Normally quite pale but eyes are bright and sparkly and a little bit of pink colour, lips are red.	Very pale, skin appears transluscent, you can see veins under skin. Eyes appear sunken and very dark shadows under eyes.
Sweating	Not particularly sweaty.	Occasionally legs appear sweaty when in bed. This is unusual because X tends to have very cold legs and feet which require regular massaging to counteract the effects of poor circulation.
Absence of contentment/ facial expression	Very contented, smiles a lot. Very sociable, likes people. Watches people and is generally happy. Likes to stroke the face of the people he knows.	Very quiet and withdrawn, not smiling, not watching people. Limited attempts to relate to others and unsociable, although still attempts to relate even when unwell or in pain.
Aggression	Not aggressive but does poke his eyes, sometimes can remove eye from socket although this doesn't tend to happen if he is distracted from poking his eye. This is thought to be a sensory self-stimulation activity, rather than a deliberate attempt to injure himself.	Bangs chin and pokes ear, this increases if he is in pain or unwell. However, action is quite subtle and understated.
Breathing	Normal breathing is quiet, occasionally has asthma requiring the use of inhaler or nebuliser.	Breathing can sound gurgly – as if he is getting a chest infection – but no evidence of this seen when further tests carried out. It sounds as if he has a build up of fluid in his throat.
Facial expression	Very smiley, happy, good eye contact, engaging.	Frowns, purses his lips – furrowed/knotted brow – makes him look like an old man.
Behaviour e.g. eating, sleeping, behaviour patterns	Sleeps well sometimes but also has bouts of wakefulness. Not restless or unhappy – just awake. Likes to listen to music when he is not asleep and is contented.	Wants to sleep all the time, but is restless. Closes eyes and drops off wherever he is. Reduced body movement, as if everything is shutting down. Likes to have someone with him.
Body tension	Quite relaxed.	No obvious changes.
Increased vocalisation	Gently vocalises from time to time, sings and giggles.	Vocalisation reduces, becomes almost completely silent and unresponsive. Responds to sudden pain by a 'growling sound'.
Crying	Not when well and comfortable.	Cries. See tears rolling down face, occasional quiet sounds and on occasion a gentle wail.
Other	Likes to be in wheelchair and able to engage with others.	Doesn't like getting in wheelchair when unwell or in pain.

Pain Picture (Gwen Moulster 2012)

Pain management recommendations

Green	Amber	Red
Sitting X up, keeping his spirits up and making him smile, talking to him. Helping X out of the wheelchair and sit up on knee. Rubbing back of X's head, rubbing his back, general massage, rubbing limbs and feet. Listening to Suzuki Violin concerto seems to relax him. Hydrotherapy. Paracetamol soluble 500mg in PEG.	As for Green plus Paracetamol 500 mg suppository when vomiting or when temperature is raised. Also given if X seems grumpy or unwell. Other interventions as for Green.	As for Amber, no other pain relief ever given.

Learning Disability Nursing at a Glance, First Edition. Edited by Bob Gates, Debra Fearns and Jo Welch. © 2015 John Wiley & Sons, Ltd. Published 2015 by John Wiley & Sons, Ltd.
Companion website: www.ataglanceseries.com/nursing/learningdisability

Pain assessment
Definition of pain

We all experience pain at times during our lives and know what action we should take when this happens. Self-reporting is recognised as the 'gold standard' for measuring our pain as it is a subjective experience and is widely acknowledged as being:

> what the experiencing person says it is, existing whenever he says it does (McCaffery, 1972).

Pain in the person with a learning disability

People with learning disabilities may find it hard to tell someone when they are in pain due to communication difficulties, yet are at increased risk of experiencing health conditions which may cause pain, for example: musculoskeletal pain from physical disabilities associated with cerebral palsy; dental caries and gum disease from poor oral hygiene and respiratory infections associated with dysphagia. If the person's pain is not recognised and its cause not treated they could be at risk of the condition progressing and possibly leading to a premature death.

For people with learning disabilities there is also the potential for 'diagnostic overshadowing' where any changes in behaviour are attributed to their learning disability and physical causes are not initially considered. Additionally, there is sometimes the misconception that people with learning disabilities have higher pain tolerance than non-learning disabled people. While some people may have impaired neural pathways others may have increased sensitivity to pain. They may also not express pain in the conventional way; possibly hitting the side of their face to indicate dental pain or earache. So they may rely on the skills of others to recognise that unusual behaviour could be a sign that they are in pain.

Having a learning disability may affect the person's ability to understand and express their pain; this does not mean that they are not experiencing discomfort, rather that carers and professionals have not picked up the cues and behaviours that are indicating pain. Evidence suggests that professionals are more likely to underestimate pain in another person and relatives may overestimate their family member's pain.

Pain assessment

Assessing if another person is in pain or the degree of pain, is not easy, and although there are a number of pain assessment tools available, their suitability would need to be considered on an individual basis, as they are not always accessible for people with learning disabilities and may offer abstract concepts that a person with a learning disability may be unable to comprehend. For example attributing a number or facial expression to pain. A comprehensive nursing assessment would provide a baseline of the individual and identify conditions which could be causing pain or likely to lead to pain. But it is important to also consider changes in physiology or behaviour that could indicate pain or discomfort.

Having established that someone is in pain, the location and possible causes also need to be established and appropriate action taken, which can be as straightforward as a change in position or may mean seeking urgent medical advice.

For people who have complex, multiple or profound disabilities, it is particularly difficult for health professionals to judge whether behavioural responses like crying are usual for the person.

One approach to the identification of possible pain is the use of a person-centred pain picture. This is developed following the completion of a family carer pain indicator. The pain picture is based on common physiological and behavioural signs of pain and the family carer's unique knowledge of the person, both when they are well and when they are in pain.

The pain picture

The pain picture can be further developed to incorporate other people's knowledge and observations of the person and provides an at a glance reference tool for the nurse, GP and others. It is designed to sit alongside the person's health action plan and health passport and can be easily updated if things change, but should be reviewed at least annually at the annual health check.

The pain picture uses a *traffic light approach* to the perceived severity of pain, with green showing a state of comfort, amber showing some discomfort and pain and red showing severe discomfort and pain. Explicit information is added to each domain about what the clinician might observe. Following the completion of the traffic light tool, commonly used interventions known to be effective for the person are identified These might include over the counter or prescribed pain relief, massage, change of position, immobilisation, mobilisation, gentle exercise, application of heat, application of ice, warm water bath, prescribed therapy and so on.

When the person is seen by the GP or hospital, the traffic light tool can help in identifying the likelihood of pain. They can then look further for causes of pain and provide timely, appropriate treatment or onward referral as needed.

In some cases there may be evidence of chronic pain. This is often misinterpreted as 'just the way the person is'; 'they always make that noise'; 'it's attention seeking behaviour'. Carers can become desensitised to the signs that someone may be in pain or discomfort. Sometimes this is because they accept information about the person passed on by other carers as being evidence based. It is important not to make assumptions and to consider could the presence of pain be a possibility? For people who are immobile unable to articulate, it should always be considered a likely possibility. The pain picture can help to identify this and enable carers to take action to reduce the effects of pain. If appropriate the person can then be referred to the pain clinic who work in partnership with the person, their family, carers, GP, learning disabilities specialists and other health and care providers to identify effective treatment and interventions and reduce the impact of pain.

The introduction of pain pictures also shows benefits for families, who can use the pain picture as a structured approach to identify changes early, enabling a speedy response and intervention and reducing the need for admission to hospital.

> Since we started using the pain picture, it has helped us by giving us a checklist to focus on to identify when our son is becoming unwell. This is really important because he is very frail and gets very sick, very quickly. When he is in pain he vomits and becomes dehydrated and nearly always ends up in hospital, this happens regularly. It is now a year since he was hospitalised and we put that down to the pain picture helping us to get pain relief and antibiotics into him promptly. (Mother of participant in Haringey Complex Health Needs Project)

41 Palliative and end-of-life care

(a) **End-of-life care**

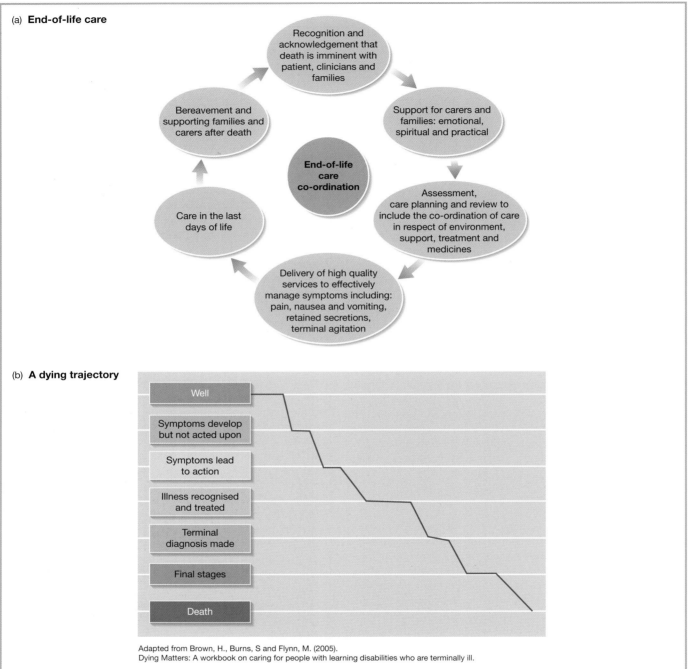

Recognition and acknowledgement that death is imminent with patient, clinicians and families

Support for carers and families: emotional, spiritual and practical

Bereavement and supporting families and carers after death

End-of-life care co-ordination

Assessment, care planning and review to include the co-ordination of care in respect of environment, support, treatment and medicines

Care in the last days of life

Delivery of high quality services to effectively manage symptoms including: pain, nausea and vomiting, retained secretions, terminal agitation

(b) **A dying trajectory**

Well

Symptoms develop but not acted upon

Symptoms lead to action

Illness recognised and treated

Terminal diagnosis made

Final stages

Death

Adapted from Brown, H., Burns, S and Flynn, M. (2005).
Dying Matters: A workbook on caring for people with learning disabilities who are terminally ill.

Introduction

The diagnosis of life-limiting illnesses often occurs late for people with a learning disability. Recognising the health deterioration of someone who has a learning disability may be difficult, especially if they are unable to say that they are feeling unwell or describe their symptoms verbally. This can lead to the potential for diagnostic overshadowing, when changes in behaviour are attributed to their learning disability and not ill health. If people are constantly living with fragile health they may regularly have periods of being unwell and seem to make a good recovery, however their general condition may be declining, and if visualised on a trajectory (see Figure (b) above) can be seen to be deteriorating. At this point, the consideration of palliative care may be appropriate.

Palliative care is the holistic care provided when curative treatment is no longer effective. It encompasses managing the physical symptoms, the person's psychosocial and spiritual needs and should also include family and friends' welfare. For people with learning disabilities this may also include care staff, who may find they have a significant and unexpected role at this time. Central to the palliative care ethos is the involvement of the people most important to the dying person and the relevant multiprofessional team; this could include the learning disability services and health facilitator.

End-of-life care is the focused care given in the last few days or hours of a person's life. People with a learning disability approaching the end of their life need high quality, accessible care that allows them to make genuine choices about their care and the changes that may be required during the end of life stages, including where they wish to die. Dignity and respect must be maintained throughout, so it is important that the right care is delivered at the right time, by the right person. Planning needs to include the consideration of the needs of families, friends, staff and other service users, and incorporate bereavement support following a death as well as support in dealing with the end-of-life issues.

All involved in the care of the individual need to develop their awareness and understanding of the end-of-life care pathway and how it relates to people who have learning disabilities.

The challenges of providing good palliative care and end of life care to people with a learning disability

- Communication: how do we tell someone with a learning disability they are dying? How do we ensure things are communicated to the person in a way they are able to understand?
- Decisions relating to palliative care should be made under the Mental Capacity Act 2005 and if the person is found to not have capacity it will become a 'best interest' decision.
- How do we ensure a person with a learning disability accesses the right service at the right time, be that learning disability services, primary care services or palliative care services?
- How do we support the range of health and social care services to communicate with the person with a learning disability who is dying?
- What is the role for learning disability services, health facilitator and/or hospital liaison nurse in the palliative care setting?
- Most people, when asked, would say they would prefer to die in their own bed with family around them. Is this any different for a person with a learning disability living in supported services?
- If someone is unable to explain their symptoms and pain, how do we ensure they are recognised and addressed?

The role of the learning disability nurse

The following are some of the key considerations to be made by learning disability nurses.

- Facilitate the early diagnosis of life threatening illnesses.
- Encourage service providers to find a sensitive way of keeping the person informed of their situation, hence giving them some control over the choices to be made.
- Try to introduce end-of-life care planning at an early point, allowing for the extra time that will undoubtedly be required to ensure understanding and involvement of the individual.
- Provide support to social care staff and/or the family of the person.
- Help others to think about the person's current living arrangements and if the person can be supported to live there until the end.
- If the person lives with other service users, encourage others to think about whether their needs require some consideration too.
- Provide support and training to hospitals and hospices who may not have experience of caring for people with learning disabilities who are dying.
- Previous bad experience of mainstream health and social care may make service users reticent to engage with those organisations which are proficient in care of the dying. Work with people to address these fears.
- Much of the expression of illness or distress will be made behaviourally by the person with a learning disability. Therefore, support will be needed to help others understand what is being communicated and how best to respond to it.
- Help carers to develop sensitive, open conversations with people with learning disabilities who are nearing the end of life which take account of the person's preferred communication style, their cognitive abilities, how well they understand the serious of their illness, death and dying.
- Ensure that people have regular access to all those professions and services required to meet the range of their end-of-life care needs – it is likely that this will include both learning disability and palliative care staff.
- A team approach which includes the service user, their family and friends as well as professionals is likely to result in the most robust advance care plan, though skilled facilitation of this is likely to be needed.
- Ensure that local healthcare professionals are aware of those approaching the end of life. Where there are mainstream systems in place to ensure consistent, high quality end-of-life care (e.g. end-of-life care register), ensure that the person is included within these.
- Liaise closely with primary care and palliative care services, ensuring that the Gold Standards Framework (a national systematic approach to providing quality in end-of-life care) is implemented effectively as appropriate.
- Liaise with the wider range of services including out-of-hours services, identification of local out-of-hours pharmacies, and inform the ambulance service of anticipated care needs and how these are likely to be expressed by someone with a learning disability.
- Understand when there is a need to formally review consideration of the best interests of the service user, and ensure that the appropriate meetings take place to make this happen involving the service user, their family, carers and other loved ones.

Summary

- There are a number of challenges facing care providers in ensuring that people with a learning disability receive high quality palliative and end-of-life care.
- Learning disability nurses have a pivotal role to play in overcoming the potential barriers.

42 Dementia in people with Down's syndrome

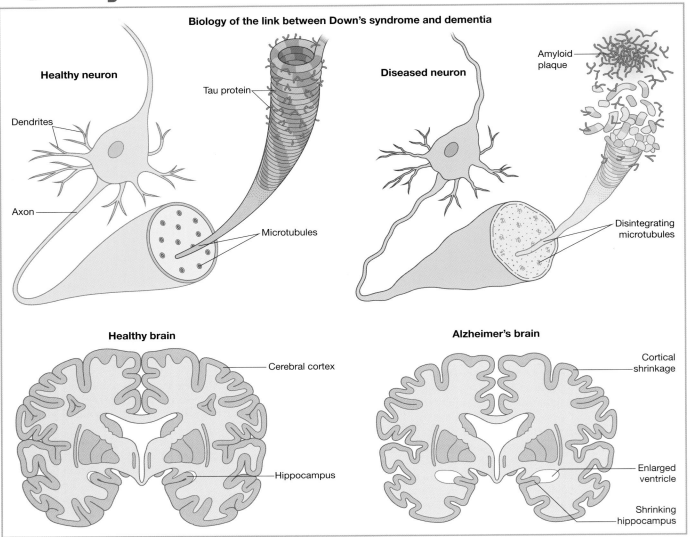

Biology of the link between Down's syndrome and dementia

Healthy neuron
- Dendrites
- Axon
- Tau protein
- Microtubules

Diseased neuron
- Amyloid plaque
- Disintegrating microtubules

Healthy brain
- Cerebral cortex
- Hippocampus

Alzheimer's brain
- Cortical shrinkage
- Enlarged ventricle
- Shrinking hippocampus

Prevalence

Dementia is 2–3 times more common in the population of people with learning disabilities than in the general population. The incidence of dementia for people with Down's syndrome is significantly greater:

- Aged 30–39 – 2%
- Aged 40–49 – 9.4%
- Aged 50–59 – 36.1%
- Aged 60–69 – 54.5%

The link between Down's syndrome and dementia

People with Down's syndrome are more likely to develop dementia (almost invariably of the Alzheimer's type) due to a known link relating to chromosome 21 (of which people with Down's syndrome have three). Amyloid is the protein that, in an insoluble form, forms the neural plaques characteristic of Alzheimer's disease. The gene coding for this protein is located on chromosome 21, and it is currently thought that this is the link accounting for the increase in risk of Alzheimer's disease in people with Down's syndrome (Figure above).

People with Down's syndrome have a rapid ageing process which is another influencing factor relating to the onset of dementia. Their life expectancy has steadily increased over the last century. In 1929 the life expectancy of a person with Down's syndrome was 9 years and currently it is estimated that over 80% of people with Down's syndrome live past 50 years of age (Kerr, 2007), meaning that the number of people who develop dementia is increasing.

Early onset and diagnosis

Early onset dementia is the term given to people who develop dementia at an earlier age than the general population, as is often the case for people with Down's syndrome. In general, people with Down's syndrome show similar symptoms to those experienced by the general population. However, due to their learning disability, there are specific issues to consider in assessing and supporting that person.

Signs and symptoms

Subtle changes in memory, mood and skills can be the first signs of dementia. For example, loss of short-term memory may result in the person forgetting to do a task or losing their property. The person's mood may also change, for example they may become agitated and more upset than they would normally be and they may lack motivation. Loss of skills may result in deterioration in the person's performance on usual tasks. The person may become confused about, for example, making a drink or getting dressed. Carers may need to prompt the person more than usual.

Such symptoms can, however, be difficult to determine, particularly when many indicators are an exaggeration of already existing behaviours and deficits due to the person's learning disability. Recognition of changes may also be delayed as they may be attributed to the persons learning disability (diagnostic overshadowing), or may occur because of a lack of knowledge and experience by the carers. Indeed, dementia can be hard to detect if others are not clear about what they are looking for. Furthermore, changes in a person's functioning may not necessarily be due to dementia but due to other conditions that may mimic symptoms of dementia. It is therefore vital that the person firstly sees their GP to exclude all other possible reasons for the changes which may include: sensory losses (both visual and hearing); thyroid functioning; depression; physical problems such as infection; environmental changes; trauma or abuse; other life events.

Assessment

It is beneficial to diagnose dementia as early as possible but it is often difficult to spot a slow decline in the abilities of someone whom carers see daily and who already has disabilities. Unfortunately, due to people moving on, staff turnover and lack of knowledge and experience by some carers, a person's historical information can be lost. It is therefore important to be aware of the person's pre-morbid state by carrying out baseline assessments regularly so that it is possible to spot changes in ability sooner rather than later. This will ultimately enable extra help and resources to be put into place as the illness progresses. Establishing a person's pre-morbid state is vital to ensure accuracy of analysis of the assessment and diagnosis and will help in supporting the person following diagnosis.

Diagnosis of dementia is not possible from a single assessment but only after careful consideration of a number of factors, which include detailed history, performance on assessments over a period of time and exclusion of all other possible reasons, as described above. There are many different formats for a baseline assessment of skills which have been developed for people who have a learning disability, with some being developed specifically for people with Down's syndrome. A range of assessment are also available that are based upon information provided by carers.

For example, Neuropsychological Assessment of Dementia on Intellectual Disabilities (NAID) and Assessment of Motor and Process skills (AMPs) can be carried out specifically with the person by learning disability health professionals. Sometimes, due to the person's low level of ability, they may be unable to carry out these assessments. In such cases different assessments can be used to gather information from carers. All of these are useful tools to gather information and to help formulate a diagnosis.

Summary

- People with Down's syndrome are living longer and hence their population is growing.
- This also means that the number of people with Down's syndrome who develop dementia will also increase; a fact that must be recognised by service providers.
- It is important not only that early diagnosis occurs, but that services are able to respond to the needs of the person with dementia.

43 Sexual health issues

(a) What do people with a learning disability worry about?

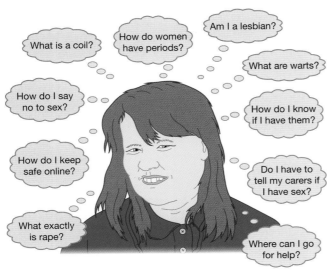

What is a coil?

How do women have periods?

Am I a lesbian?

What are warts?

How do I say no to sex?

How do I know if I have them?

How do I keep safe online?

Do I have to tell my carers if I have sex?

What exactly is rape?

Where can I go for help?

(c) Staff need training too

In order for the staff to support people with learning disability with their sexual health they need training too

(b) Working within the Sexual Offences Act 2003

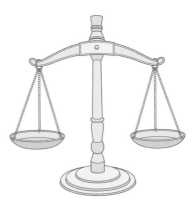

This is important legislation and affects the sex education which may be offered to someone with a mental disorder.

Care workers' offences:

'It is an offence to watch someone else taking part in sexual activity – including looking at images such as videos, photos, or webcams – for the purpose of your own sexual gratification. It is not intended that this should prevent care workers from providing legitimate sex education with an approved care plan.'

Sexual health

Introduction

The Sexual Health and HIV Strategy (DoH, 2001) proposed the following:

Sexual health is an important part of physical and mental health. It is a key part of our identity as human beings together with the fundamental human rights to privacy, a family life and living free from discrimination. Essential elements of good sexual health are equitable relationships and sexual fulfilment with access to information and services to avoid the risk of unintended pregnancy, illness or disease.

It also encompasses social wellbeing in relation to sexuality, sexual relationships which are pleasurable, experiences that are not frightening or abusive. People with learning disability (PwLD) need to have correct information about the many issues involved, including names for their bodies, services and where to go for help. They have lots of questions that sometimes need different mediums and time to be addressed, they need confidence in the people that are helping them and to trust that they have the correct and up-to-date information (Figure (a) above).

The Royal College of Nursing (RCN, 2000) recognises that sexuality and sexual health promotion/education are part of holistic care and developed a sexual health strategy to guide nurses in this area. This feeds in to the wider teenage pregnancy and sexual health strategy (DoH, 1998).

What is sex education?

This can sometimes be called sex and relationships education and helps PwLD to raise awareness, collect information, be empowered to form views and ideas, learn about emotions, sexual identity, relationships, good and bad touching, keeping safe, contraception, sexually transmitted infections, intimacy and sex.

Sex education is about giving opportunities and helping to develop skills so that choices are recognised, decisions are then made based on correct information which in turn builds confidence and competence when acting on these choices. This helps to protect people with learning disabilities from abuse, exploitation, unintended pregnancies, sexually transmitted infections and aids in developing healthy coping strategies in their relationships.

These skills that are developed are life-long skills. Relationships are built on good communication, listening, negotiation; knowledge and awareness and making decisions based on correct information and identifying sources and agencies of where to go for help and when they need help (Figure (b) above).

The role of the learning disability nurse

For PwLD, sex education can be offered at any stage in their life where it is necessary and important for them to have this information as they are ready to receive it, and correctly pitched for them. Staff must be aware of the Sexual Offences Act 2003 and keep in mind their limitations when providing sex education. They also need to have training for themselves in order to empower PwLD (Figure (c) above).

Sex education topics could include sessions covering hygiene, emotions, good and bad touching, different types of relationships, keeping safe (to include internet), intimacy, sex and sexual health, contraception, sexually transmitted infections, sex and the law and access to sexual health agencies.

The social networks of people with learning disabilities

People with learning disabilities are likely to:
- Have social networks that are smaller than those of members of the general population.
- Have proportionately fewer friends than people *without* learning disabilities.
- Nominate a large number of service providers as being members of their social network.
- Rely on family members for the provision of *emotional* support.
- Be relatively isolated within the general community.
- Experience social relationships that are non-reciprocal (i.e. not characterised by 'give-and-take') and seen as 'passive recipients' of support.

44 Postural care

Protection of body shape

Postural care is a gentle, passive form of physical therapy used to protect a person's body shape. It is effective if it is used consistently over a 24-hour period. It is important to recognise the significance of night time when considering postural care due to the significant amount of time that people spend in bed.

- On average a child will spend 1140 hours of the year in school, slightly longer if an adult is at work.
- If they go to bed at 9 pm and get up at 7 am they will be in bed for 3650 hours of the year.
- Many people with a complex disability will spend longer than this in bed.
- Being physically active during the day is very important but good positioning is vital if a person is to remain symmetrical.
- People who provide an individual's hands-on care are the key to good postural care.

Body shape distortion occurs gradually over time. Common examples of body shape distortion include hip subluxation or dislocation, pelvic obliquity and scoliosis.

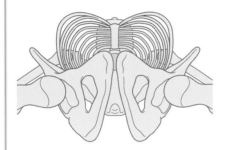

Chest symmetry

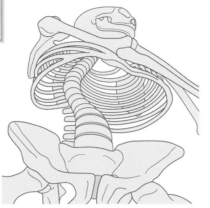

Clockwise rotational distortion

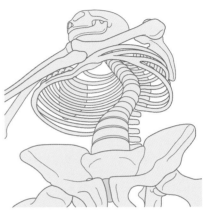

Anticlockwise rotational distortion

How do you know if the person needs postural care?

- If they find it difficult to change position independently, regardless of their age or diagnosis, you need to consider postural care.
- Consider the positions that the person is able to adopt and whether these are destructive or supported.
- Within a 24 hour period assess the likely impact of these positions. Very short periods of time in destructive postures, for example when a person is using a hoist, will have less impact compared with long periods of time, for example when a person is asleep in bed. This will be heavily influenced by the quality and appropriateness of the equipment the person has access to.

Commonly used terms and concepts to be aware of

- Destructive postures – postures in which the skeleton, internal organs and muscle tone can be damaged. Usually these are asymmetric postures in which some joints will be stressed.
- Supported postures – postures in which the skeleton and joints are supported in neutral, comfortable positions, internal capacity of the chest and abdomen are protected.
- Primitive pathological reflexes – in a newborn baby, primitive reflexes can be seen to influence the way they move. As the child develops, these primitive reflexes are replaced by postural reflexes which help to support the child to move against gravity and to produce more complicated movement. Some children retain these primitive reflexes if their balance and core stability does not develop.
- Postural reflexes support control of balance, stability and movement, normally replacing primitive reflexes as more mature patterns of movement develop.
- Muscle tone – the state of readiness of muscles to contract, relax, coordinate and stabilise. High tone (hypertonic) the muscle is too tight, low tone (hypotonic) the muscle is too loose.
- Prone – the word used to describe lying on your stomach. Supine – the word used to describe lying on your back.
- Symmetrical supine lying – the position in which the heavy parts of the body, the spine, back of the pelvis, shoulder blades and the back of the head are best supported. In this position the softer more vulnerable parts of the body such as the front of the chest are less likely to be damaged.
- Side lying – a position in which rotational forces acting on the body will inevitably cause damage. This position is used for short periods to support the development of function but wherever possible should be avoided for long periods of time.

Equipment used to protect body shape

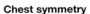

Wheelchairs

Alternative or comfortable seating

Bath and shower seats

Specialist car seats

Orthotics

Standing frames

v

Sleep systems

Learning Disability Nursing at a Glance, First Edition. Edited by Bob Gates, Debra Fearns and Jo Welch. © 2015 John Wiley & Sons, Ltd. Published 2015 by John Wiley & Sons, Ltd.
Companion website: www.ataglanceseries.com/nursing/learningdisability

Postural care

Postural care is used to protect a person's body shape. Very young children rarely have distorted body shapes as distortion occurs gradually over a long period of time. Gravity and destructive postures conspire to distort body shape in a predictable and avoidable way. Those people who provide hands-on day-to-day care need to be supported to understand how to provide gentle postural care over the 24-hour period.

Assessment

If the person you support finds it difficult to change position independently you need to think about whether they need to use postural care. The Mansfield Checklist can be used to help identify people that are at risk of body shape distortion:

- Does the person stay in a limited number of positions?
- Do the person's knees seem to be drawn to one side? Inwards? Outwards?
- Are the person's arms and hands in a position in which they could function easily?
- Does the person's head seem to turn mainly to one side?
- Does the person's body tend to extend backwards? Flex forwards? Fall to the right or to the left?

Measurement of body symmetry

Validated, standardised and non-invasive measurement of body symmetry provides an accurate baseline of the symmetry of the body. It is used to determine the therapeutic forces that are required either to maintain symmetry or to restore the body to a symmetrical, balanced posture. The measures are called The Goldsmith Indices of Body Symmetry and are used alongside other information, such as the condition of a person's hips, to determine the success of therapeutic intervention.

Use of equipment

There is a very wide range of equipment that may be used to provide people with comfortable support and to protect their body symmetry.

- Tilt in space seating enables both the seat and back to be tilted forward or backwards without altering the angle at the hips, this is used in combination with recline to offer a range of seating positions over time.
- Recline allows for the angle of the hip to be opened which reduces the destructive impact of gravity on a person in an upright posture. Recline also increases the internal capacity of the abdomen and thorax so enabling improved function of the internal organs.
- Modular seating comprises a seating base with a range of moveable parts which can be selected and positioned according to the person's needs.
- Moulded seating comprises of a seating base which is moulded around the individual person's body. This may enable those with severe body shape distortion to be able to access mobility, but is far less flexible and dynamic than a modular system.
- Seating may be used to support particular activities, such as bath, shower and car seats.
- Standing frames are used to enable a person to be supported to bear weight, the person may not necessarily be in an upright position. If the person shows any signs of pain or distress, if their hips are damaged or their body is rotated careful consideration should be given as to the intended benefits of standing.
- Orthotics such as callipers, splints and braces may be prescribed to provide long-term, gentle support. Short-term stretching of limbs to maintain muscle length and range of movement is not recommended within NICE Guidelines.
- Lycra suits can provide support and reduce high tone in order to enable the individual to function more easily.
- Sleep systems offer support for the person in lying. They may be used during the day but are generally used at night and have made a significant contribution to protecting body shape. It is widely acknowledged that a 24-hour approach to postural care is essential and since positioning people at night time has become widely used the therapeutic benefits have been found to be extremely positive.

Careful consideration must be given to:

1 Why a particular piece of equipment is being used.
2 Are the person and those using the equipment happy with it?
3 Have the first circle of support been trained in the safe use of the equipment?
4 Is the equipment well maintained, does it fit, is it appropriate?
5 What is the intended benefit for any given piece of equipment and how will this be demonstrated?

Safety planning

Particular consideration must be given to the safety of night time positioning. People may well be either asleep or tired, there may are fewer people around and fewer opportunities to monitor the person's wellbeing. The following list is not exhaustive but highlights common safety considerations:

- Is the person happy?
- Does the person have epilepsy?
- Can they breathe safely?
- Are they comfortable with regard to temperature?
- Are there any new pressure areas resulting from a change in body position?
- Are there any problems with circulation?
- Does the person use enteral feeding at night?
- Does the person have reflux?
- Are continence issues resolved?
- Are there any other issues which need to be thought about in order to make sure that changes of position will be introduced safely and gently?

Summary
- Postural care is a person-centred 24-hour approach that has been shown to both protect and restore body shape, muscle tone and quality of life. It is essential that the person and their first circle of support are well trained to self-manage this long-term aspect of healthcare.

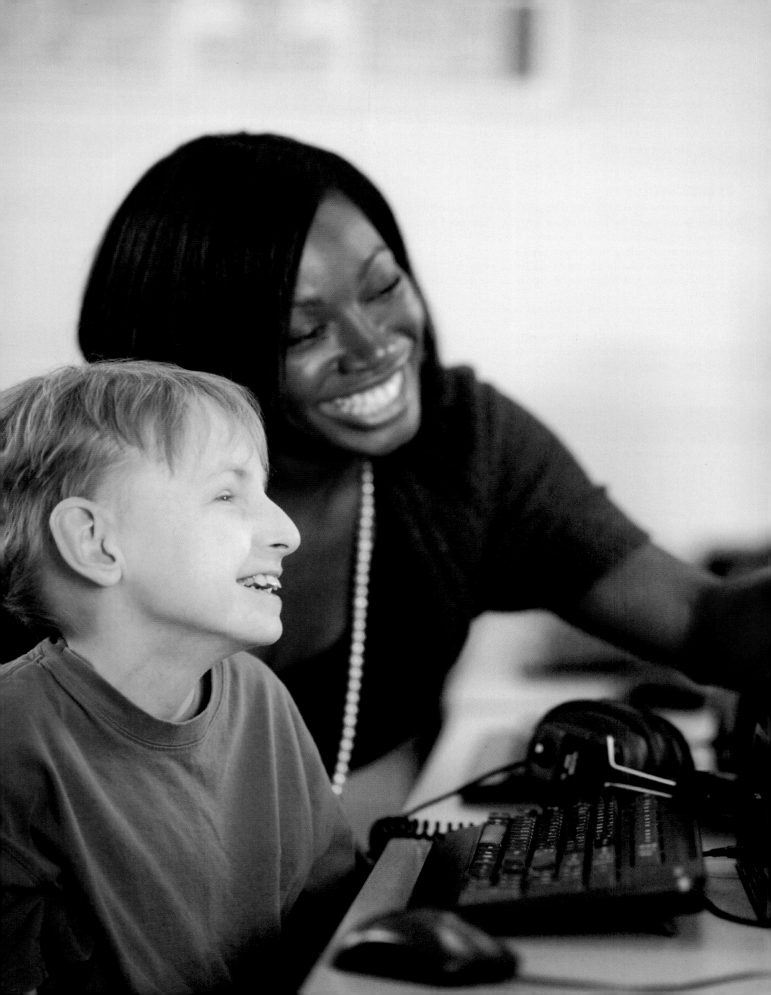

Older people with a learning disability

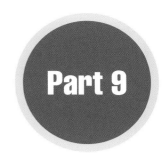

Part 9

Chapters

45 **Older people with a learning disability** 104

46 **Dementia care** 106

47 **The Mental State Examination** 108

Don't forget to visit the companion website for this book at www.ataglanceseries.com/nursing/learningdisability to do some practice cases on these topics.

45 Older people with a learning disability

Test	Frequency	Age	Gender
Cervical screening	Every 3 years	Up to 65	Female
Breast screening	Every 3 years	50–65 (and beyond if had previous abnormal result)	Female
Bowel cancer	Every 2 years	65–70 (can be requested post-70)	Both
AAA (Abdominal Aortic Aneurysm)	Once	In the 65th year	Male
Eye test and screening for glaucoma	Every two years Every year	Aged 60–70 Over 70	Both
Diabetic retinopathy screening	Annually for those with diabetes		Both

Older people with a learning disability

Along with the rest of the population, people with a learning disabilities are living longer than ever before, although the average lifespan remains considerably shorter than the general population with a higher level of preventable premature deaths. As people age, their health and social care needs are likely to increase or change, even people who previously had very little contact with health or social services will start to use them.

Definitions

Older people are usually thought to be those over the state retirement age, however, many studies have suggested this should be much younger for people with learning disabilities (i.e. over 50 years or over 60 years) as a result of the conditions associated with learning disability that also cause premature ageing. Common characteristics associated with old age are often used to classify people with learning disabilities, rather than chronological age, and it is worth bearing in mind that individuals with learning disabilities will be as diverse in their experiences of old age and their needs for services as the general population.

Bio-psychosocial model of ageing

Any model in relation to ageing needs to ensure a holistic approach, recognising and responding to the different aspects of a person's life. As with childhood, adolescence, adulthood and middle age, the biological, psychological and social aspects of life influence and impact on each other to determine the health of an individual in old age.

The role for learning disability nursing

Identifying and meeting health needs

Learning disability nurses (LDNs) need to be aware of the physical health needs associated with ageing, such as sensory impairment, dementias, respiratory disease, heart disease, stroke, increased likelihood of certain cancers, osteoporosis, continence changes, changes to mobility, skin integrity, and so on. Identifying these health needs can be improved through the use of screening and assessment tools and by ensuring that people with learning disabilities are included in screening programmes aimed at older people (see Table above).

Screening tests are commonly used for older people (e.g. prostate cancer, cholesterol, thyroid function, anaemia, kidney disease, osteoporosis, hearing) but rely on people reporting symptoms to their GP or practice nurse, it is therefore essential that LDNs can recognise these symptoms and encourage and support people to use primary care services.

In addition to the ordinary health needs of old age, there are some of specific relevance to people with learning disabilities that LDNs need to be able to identify and meet. The leading cause of death for people with learning disabilities is respiratory disease, often exacerbated by late diagnosis and treatment. LDNs need to be able to recognise early signs and symptoms to facilitate early treatment and prevent premature death. Similarly, dementias are often not diagnosed in the early stages and therefore are not eligible for the same range of treatment options. In addition, some conditions and syndromes have health implications as people age that need to be accounted for in care plans (e.g. reduced skin integrity in people with Down's syndrome).

Some Community Teams for people with learning disabilities have developed care pathways for specific conditions associated with older age, such as dementia, which provide evidence-based guidance for identification and interventions for these conditions.

The mental health needs of older people can be easily overlooked, particularly in people with limited communication, but this is known to be an area of increased need in older people. LDNs can help to identify signs of depression and other mental health needs as a person ages and, along with the wider multidisciplinary team, work on strategies to prevent these occurring or reduce the impact. It is important to remember that as people age, hectic daily activities are not necessarily wanted, and activity needs to be balanced with sufficient intellectual stimulation, physical activity and periods of rest.

Reducing health inequalities

A key role for LDNs is promoting the use of reasonable adjustments to reduce health inequalities for people with learning disabilities. For older people, this means working closely with primary care services to ensure that people are included in screening and immunisation programmes (e.g. flu vaccinations) and supporting them to make changes to the way they deliver those services if necessary.

It also includes training and education events with parents, carers, primary care and hospital staff to increase awareness of 'diagnostic overshadowing' and how to avoid it; assessment of mental capacity as people age; pain assessment and management; planning for end of life. In terms of mental wellbeing, LDNs also need to consider the psychological implications of ageing and work with services such as bereavement counsellors to ensure they are available to people with learning disabilities.

In order to reduce health inequalities, LDNs need to identify health and social care services that are involved in the care of older people and ensure that those services are aware of services for people with learning disabilities and the availability of training and support.

Promoting social inclusion

Improved access to health services and better health outcomes will enable older people to maintain social relationships, participate in activities, and remain in their own homes longer, which all contribute to social inclusion. However, one of the biggest challenges for LDNs working with older people can be living arrangements.

A significant percentage of people with learning disabilities live with parents or relatives and, as they get older, so are their parents and relatives. This brings challenges in terms of their fitness and abilities to maintain a caring role, possibly in the face of more demanding caring needs and anxieties about where a person will live if/when they are not able to care for them or die themselves. LDNs need to be able to raise these concerns with care and compassion and support people with transition planning as the health and wellbeing of carers or the person with a learning disability deteriorate. In some circumstances advocacy services can be very helpful.

For people living in residential or supported living services, there is also a need for transition planning or planning for the future. Other people sharing the residence and staff teams are likely to experience grief as people's needs change and they have to move on, or as health deteriorates and death occurs. LDNs have an important role to play in supporting peers and staff teams in managing expectations as people age and enabling them to maintain relationships for as long as possible. This could involve staff training (e.g. on how to prevent pressure ulcers) or liaising with the wider multidisciplinary team to assist with psychological support, physiotherapy, adaptations to the environment or social work to examine alternative options.

As people age, it is quite common for spirituality to become more important to them and LDNs need to be aware of this and facilitate opportunities for people to express this. This may mean working with local religious groups to support people to be included in different forms of religious observation. Or it may involve working with the person to make sense of their life and place in the world, for instance by completing a life story, a memory box or a family tree.

Another important aspect of social inclusion for older people with learning disabilities is their involvement in cultural practices around the death of a relative or friend. Research has shown that excluding people from such practices (e.g. funerals, wakes) can lead to psychological or mental health problems. The view can be put forward that such occasions will be too distressing for a person with a learning disability and the role of a LDN is to advocate for that person while maintaining care and compassion for other people involved. This may involve assessing the person's understanding and providing information in a way that is meaningful to them so that they can make a decision about the extent to which they are involved and supporting them with that.

46 Dementia care

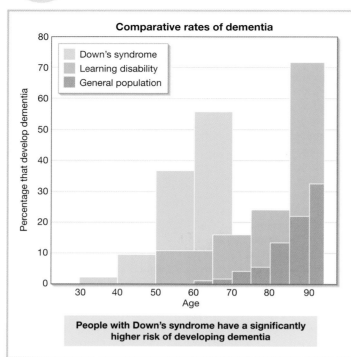

Comparative rates of dementia

- Down's syndrome
- Learning disability
- General population

Percentage that develop dementia / Age

People with Down's syndrome have a significantly higher risk of developing dementia

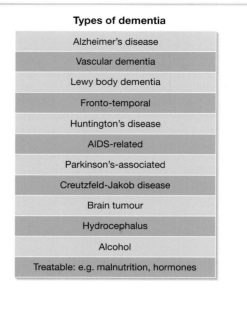

Types of dementia

Alzheimer's disease
Vascular dementia
Lewy body dementia
Fronto-temporal
Huntington's disease
AIDS-related
Parkinson's-associated
Creutzfeld-Jakob disease
Brain tumour
Hydrocephalus
Alcohol
Treatable: e.g. malnutrition, hormones

What is dementia?

Dementia is a global term describing a group of diseases that affect the brain and leads to progressive loss of brain tissue. It is a progressive and usually gradual decline and can affect language abilities, emotions and behaviour. It is often not diagnosed, especially in people with learning disabilities, because the symptoms can be subtle and develop slowly, symptoms can often be wrongly attributed to the learning disability, and carers can often 'compensate' for the person's cognitive deficits (diagnostic overshadowing).

Prevalence

It is estimated that there are 570 000 people with dementia in England, giving an approximate number of 11 400 people with a learning disability and dementia (based on the research figures that approximately 2% of the population have a learning disability). This needs to be weighed against the recognition that dementia is a condition which is greatly under-diagnosed. It is thought that only a third of people with dementia actually receive a formal diagnosis. This statistic will be more significant for people with a learning disability due to the additional diagnosis issues relating to the overshadowing of the dementia by the learning disability. Hence, the figures given here can be viewed as no more than a general estimation.

Stages of dementia

- Early Stage – often categorised by subtle changes in memory, mood and skills.

- Middle Stage – increased forgetfulness, disorientation, mood changes, slowness withdrawal, and sleep problems.
- Late Stage – 24-hour care, reduced mobility increased physical health problems, reduced skills in all areas and memory loss.

Difficulties of early diagnosis

The clinical picture depends on the type of disease process, areas of the brain most affected and the individual. The onset of symptoms is insidious and symptoms can be variable. They are often not recognised or acknowledged by carers, and hence not reported to healthcare professionals in a reliable way. Symptoms may also be due to other causes and a full assessment of an individual's health and social needs is required. Only once all other potential causes of the presentation have been explored and addressed, can a diagnosis of dementia be concluded.

Supporting people with dementia
Communication

Good communication is at the heart of all effective therapeutic interventions. This entails being aware of non-verbal cues and speaking appropriately in line with the person's level of comprehension, sensory abilities and culture. The written word or pictures may also be helpful. It is important to appreciate that some people may have sensory deficits, and regular vision and hearing tests should be carried out. Working with people with learning disability and dementia requires flexibility because their abilities may fluctuate and this needs to be accommodated.

Learning Disability Nursing at a Glance, First Edition. Edited by Bob Gates, Debra Fearns and Jo Welch. © 2015 John Wiley & Sons, Ltd. Published 2015 by John Wiley & Sons, Ltd.
Companion website: www.ataglanceseries.com/nursing/learningdisability

Maintaining skills

The dementia process will affect how the person is able to carry out tasks. The emphasis is to maintain a person's skills and independence for as long as possible, not to teach them new skills. Aids and adaptations can help in maintaining skills. Activities should be stimulating, predictable and failure free. Tasks should not be time limited and should take place in a calm environment free of distraction. When exploring appropriate activities, it is also important to consider the right level of stimulation and challenge for the individual. The complexity of activity and level of engagement will change. However, it should not be assumed that the person with dementia does not retain abilities to perform an activity. Individualised and creative ways need to be explored to maximise the use of an individual's strengths well into the later stages of dementia. Social networks, voluntary services, communities, and health and social services can play an important role in socially including people and maximising independence at all stages of illness.

Memory aids such as calendars, diaries, schedules of daily routine, memory books or electronic devices are also useful to aid individual's routine in the earlier stages of dementia.

Therapeutic interventions

People with dementia are likely to respond differently to the variety of psychological and pharmacological management strategies. It is important to know the range of interventions and which ones may be most appropriate for an individual taking into account their learning disability, and to understand how to recognise whether an intervention is helping. Promoting independence and maintaining function are vital aspects of treatment and care.

Reminiscent work and life stories

Memories help us to know who we are. Reminiscing reminds us of the world and our identity and can be a pleasurable activity. Knowing the person is important for those caring for the people with dementia. Reminiscent work can help to maintain communication and cognitive processes. Developing life stories can help the person to remember their life through pictures and objects and can be an aid to engaging the person through communication while helping to ensure that their history is not lost.

Environment

A dementia-friendly environment will help to maintain independence. A person with dementia needs to live in a familiar environment with people known to them. Introducing drastic changes to a person's life will be detrimental to them. Environments should be stress free, calm and designed with a person's sensory and other problems in mind. Pictures and signs can help the person to find their way around their home. Consideration for reflective surfaces needs to be made as people may not recognise their reflection. The environment should be organised in a way that makes it easy to know where things are kept. Choices should be limited to avoid confusion and anxiety.

Pharmacological interventions

Once a diagnosis has been determined, drugs can be prescribed to slow the progression of the disease. However, family and support staff should be made aware that they will not cure the dementia, only delay the progression, and the medication will eventually need to be stopped. The main drugs currently in use are Donepezil, Galantamine, Rivastigmine and Memantine.

The importance of keeping healthy

People with learning disabilities and dementia will continue to have additional health needs, some of which will be directly linked to the progression of the dementia. There is a high risk that epilepsy may develop in the late stages of dementia. Depression is often seen during the early stages. Pain may go undiagnosed due to communication difficulties. General poor health, if not diagnosed and treated, will further impact upon the person's wellbeing.

Summary

- People with a learning disability are at an increased risk of developing dementia.
- Assessments and diagnosis of dementia is more difficult for this group of people due to the pre-existing cognitive impairments.
- Interventions may include psychological and pharmacological treatments.
- However, providing supportive care that encourages patients to maintain as much independent functioning as possible is perhaps as important as any specific interventions for cognitive symptoms.

47 # The Mental State Examination

The Mental State Examination: what is assessed, and making provision for the people with a learning disability

Appearance and behaviour

- Consider the individual's appearance: do they appear physically well/unwell? Have they attended to personal care needs? What are they wearing? Is this appropriate to the weather and situation? Are they kempt/unkempt?

- For people with a learning disability bear in mind they may require support to get dressed and attend to personal care needs.

- If they do receive support with personal care, ask about their response to that personal care and whether there was engagement, reluctance or refusal on the day of assessment.

- Observe the individual's behaviour: consider the level of motor activity; is there evidence of psychomotor agitation (increased movement) or psychomotor retardation (slowing down of movement)? Is the individual engaged in the assessment? Are they making eye contact? Are there any abnormal movements? Is there evidence of side-effects from antipsychotic medication?

- Bear in mind the individual's learning disability and any behaviours that may be associated with that, for example stereotypical movements such as rocking and poor eye contact may be associated with autism or learning disability.

Perception

- There are three broad types of perceptual disturbance: hallucinations, pseudo-hallucinations and illusions.

Cognition

- This section is composed of structured tests as well as unstructured observations.

Insight

- Insight is the individual's understanding of their mental illness and ranges from denial to full understanding.

- The level of the individual's learning disability and cognitive functioning must be taken into account as insight may be difficult to assess.

Speech

- Assess rate, tone and volume, including pressure of speech (high volume, rapid speech which is difficult to interrupt).

- Assess the content and quality of speech and whether it is logical or incoherent. Is speech repetitive? Is there evidence of neologising?

- Assessing the speech of people with a learning disability may be difficult because of communication difficulties. Although this section of the MSE is based upon verbal communication, it may be necessary to consider other methods of communication used by the individual.

- Knowledge of the individual's usual communication style is important, including use of repetitive words or specific words/phrases that are unique to them.

Mood and affect

- When assessing mood it is beneficial to also identify physiological symptoms such as dry mouth, palpitations, sweating and tremor: these may be linked to symptoms of anxiety or poor sleep pattern, withdrawal from usual activities and changes in libido or appetite.

- Assess the stability of mood and congruence.

- It may be difficult for people with a learning disability to understand their mood or describe how they are feeling, so it is beneficial to also obtain information from a reliable informant.

Thoughts

- Identify whether there is evidence of negative thought patterns, suicidal ideation, delusions, depersonalisation, obsessions, compulsions, rumination and abnormal beliefs.

- This may be particularly difficult to assess for people with a learning disability who may find it hard to express and communicate these thoughts; the assessor may need to obtain information from informant interviews and observations.

- Be mindful that people with a learning disability may have less grandiose delusions. It is important to consider delusions with respect to the individual's level of functioning.

People with a learning disability experience the same range of psychiatric illness as people without a learning disability. In addition to this, research also reports that people with a learning disability experience a higher prevalence of psychiatric illness than the population as a whole. It is therefore important for learning disability nurses to be able to recognise the symptoms or characteristics that may be indicative of mental ill health. Nurses must be able to undertake an accurate assessment of a person's health, including mental health, in order to inform nursing diagnosis and contribute information for medical diagnosis to inform care planning and interventions.

The assessment of psychiatric illness in people with learning disabilities faces many challenges. Self-reporting of symptoms can be reduced dependent on the individual's level of learning disability

and cognitive and verbal communication skills. The nurse may also be reliant upon third-party information from carers and there can be an overlap between the presentation of symptoms for psychiatric disorders, learning disability, behavioural phenotypes and manifestation of physical ill health. It is therefore essential that a bio-psychosocial model to understanding health is applied to ensure thorough and accurate assessment. This should include consideration of the risk factors that may predispose the individual to mental illness, potential triggers to mental illness and on-going factors that are exacerbating the individual's mental health.

Due to the complexity of assessing psychiatric illness for people with a learning disability there are a range of validated tools to support the assessment process. These include specific checklists such as the Glasgow Anxiety Scale (GAS) and Glasgow Depression Scale

Learning Disability Nursing at a Glance, First Edition. Edited by Bob Gates, Debra Fearns and Jo Welch. © 2015 John Wiley & Sons, Ltd. Published 2015 by John Wiley & Sons, Ltd.
Companion website: www.ataglanceseries.com/nursing/learningdisability

(GDS) and further assessment tools and guidance including the PAS-ADD (Psychiatric Assessment Schedules for Adults with Developmental Disabilities) and DC-LD (Diagnostic criteria for psychiatric disorders for people with Learning Disabilities). These tools support the nurse and other practitioners in assessing the presentation and symptoms of psychiatric illness. One important tool for assessing psychiatric illness is the Mental State Examination (MSE). This, alongside a good medical and psychiatric history, will support the nurse in gathering the information required to make a formulation. The MSE assesses the individual's mental state at the time of assessment, it is a snapshot of the patients mental state at that given time and therefore differentiates from the psychiatric history.

The Mental State Examination requires the person undertaking the assessment to consider a range of factors including: appearance, behaviour, speech, mood, thought, perception, cognition and insight. The MSE will begin as soon as the practitioner meets the individual. When undertaking MSE for people with a learning disability it is important to consider the individual's ability to self-report symptoms and to identify reliable informants, as reliance simply on informants or self-report can reduce the accuracy of the assessment. It is also important to recognise that the presentation of symptoms may be different for people with a learning disability due to their cognitive functioning, levels of support and expression of symptoms. The MSE can fluctuate from day to day or even over a number of hours; therefore, it is helpful to gather as much information as possible about the MSE when undertaking the individuals' psychiatric history.

Appearance and behaviour

Consider the individual's appearance, and the factors outlined in the Table above. Also, you should observe the individual's behaviour during the assessment, and consider the level of motor activity. Whilst assessing behavioural presentation during the MSE, the assessor must consider the individual's learning disability and any behaviours that may be associated with this, for example stereotypical movements such as rocking and poor eye contact may be associated with autism or learning disability.

Speech

See the Table above for what to assess. Assessment of speech is particularly difficult for people with a learning disability due to communication difficulties. This section of the MSE is based upon verbal communication but the assessor may need to consider other methods of communication used by the individual. Knowledge of the individual's usual communication is important and consideration of their learning disability is essential as it may be common for them to use repetitive words or to have specific phrases or words that are unique to them.

Mood and affect

Assessment of mood refers to the emotions expressed by the individual or observed by the assessor through behaviour. This may be low mood or elevated mood. When assessing mood it is beneficial to identify physiological symptoms alongside feelings and emotions. The stability of mood and congruence should also be assessed.

Thoughts

Thoughts relate to how an individual thinks and how they process information and situations. Identify whether there is evidence of negative thought patterns; this is particularly difficult to assess for people with a learning disability who may find it difficult to express and communicate these thoughts.

Perception

Perception in the context of the MSE is any sensory experience.

A **hallucination** is defined as a sensory perception in the absence of any external stimulus, and is experienced by the person as being real.

An **illusion** is a false sensory experience, often experienced as being false by the person.

A **pseudo hallucination** is experienced in internally (for example, hearing 'voices in my head') and is regarded as similar to fantasy.

Cognition

This section of the MSE covers the person's level of alertness, orientation, concentration, memory, visual-spatial awareness and language skills.

Insight

Insight is the individual's understanding of their mental illness. It may range from a complete denial of having a mental illness to a complete understanding of the effect of mental illness upon the person themselves, as well as upon others, and with an acceptance or refusal of treatment.

Challenges

There are specific challenges in carrying out an MSE with people with learning disabilities (see Table above). The person carrying out the assessment needs to examine and clarify the person's use of words to describe mood, thought content or perceptions, as words may be used uniquely and have a different meaning to the ones understood by the person carrying out the exam. In this instance, tools such as play materials, puppets, art materials or diagrams may be used to assist recall and explain their experiences.

Summary

- Nurses may need to gather information from carers as well as the person with a learning disability to be able to gain a more accurate picture of the overall physical and mental health needs being presented.
- There are a range of tools available for assessment, but the Mental State Examination provides a 'snapshot' of the person's mental state at that given time.
- It is also important to recognise that the presentation of symptoms may be different for people with a learning disability due to their cognitive functioning, levels of support and expression of symptoms.

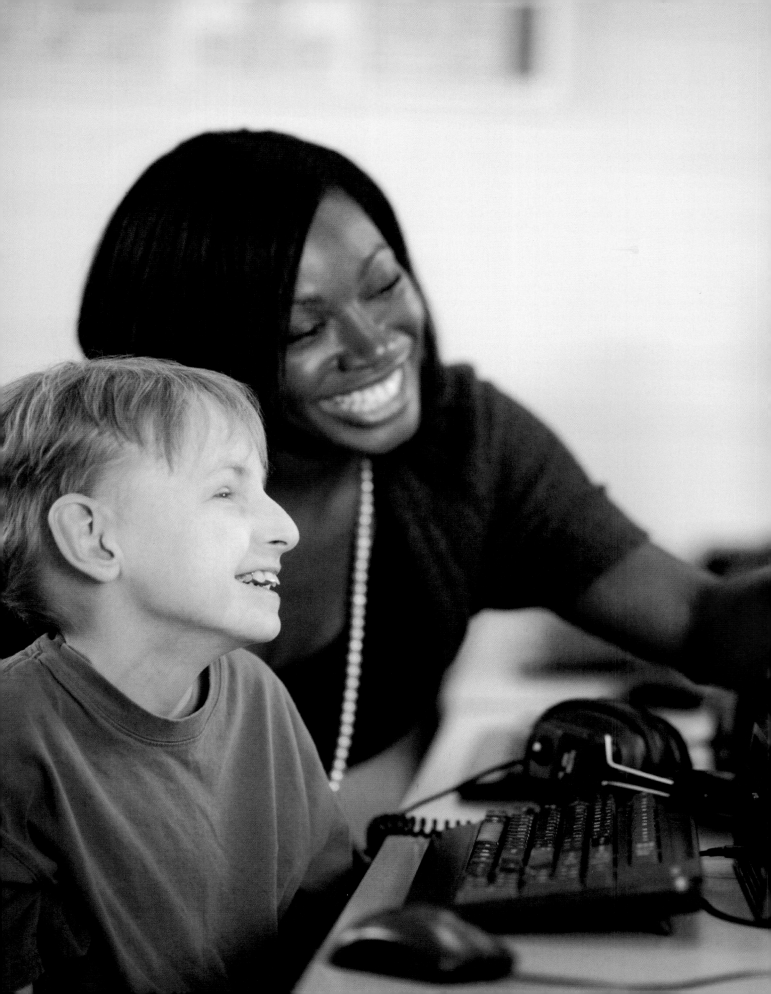

Medication

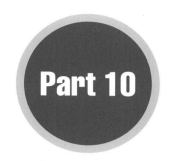

Part 10

Chapters

48 Antidepressant and antipsychotic drugs 112
49 Antiepileptic drugs 114
50 Nurse prescribing 116
51 Drug calculations 118

Don't forget to visit the companion website for this book at
www.ataglanceseries.com/nursing/learningdisability to
do some practice cases on these topics.

48 Antidepressant and antipsychotic drugs

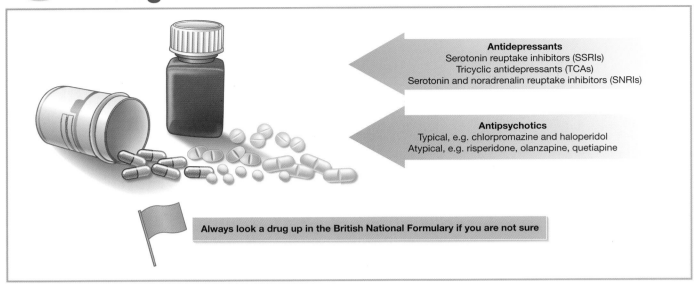

Antidepressants
Serotonin reuptake inhibitors (SSRIs)
Tricyclic antidepressants (TCAs)
Serotonin and noradrenalin reuptake inhibitors (SNRIs)

Antipsychotics
Typical, e.g. chlorpromazine and haloperidol
Atypical, e.g. risperidone, olanzapine, quetiapine

Always look a drug up in the British National Formulary if you are not sure

Antidepressants and antipsychotics

People with a learning disability are up to four times more likely to be suffering from a mental illness. Psychiatrists (and sometimes GPs) will often use antidepressant medication or antipsychotic medication to treat mental illness, in conjunction with input from the rest of the multidisciplinary team. All the medications discussed below are started at a low dose and gradually increased to an effective dose.

Antidepressant medication

Antidepressant medication can be used for the treatment of anxiety disorders, including obsessional thoughts and behaviours, as well as depression. In people with a learning disability, they can also be used for self-injurious behaviour. It can take up to eight weeks for an improvement to be seen after starting someone on antidepressant medication. The most commonly used are serotonin reuptake inhibitors (SSRIs), but other classes of antidepressant include tricyclic antidepressants (TCAs), serotonin and noradrenalin reuptake inhibitors (SNRIs) and a few others which are less commonly used.

SSRIs

Drugs in this class are fluoxetine, sertraline, citalopram, escitalopram, paroxetine and fluvoxamine. It is most likely that a person will be taking one of the first four drugs, although some patients who have been on medication for a significant period of time could also be taking paroxetine or fluvoxamine.

SSRIs are generally safe and well-tolerated. The commonest side-effects occur mostly in the first two weeks and include restlessness, anxiety, nausea, diarrhoea and indigestion. These tend to settle with time. Serious, but less common, side-effects may be an increase in suicidal feelings, difficulty urinating or confusion.

Tricyclic antidepressants

Tricyclic antidepressants are older drugs with more side-effects. The most commonly used is amitryptiline, but imipramine and clomipramine are also sometimes used. They are also used in low dose for chronic pain and sometimes for difficulty with sleeping. The common side-effects of these drugs are dry mouth, sedation, constipation, difficulty urinating and dizziness. The dose is usually increased very slowly over time because of the side-effects. They are extremely dangerous in overdose.

SNRIs

The most commonly used drug is venlafaxine. This is a very effective treatment for anxiety and depression, but should be prescribed by psychiatrists rather than GPs. It is only tried after at least one other antidepressant has been tried. It can cause raised blood pressure and cardiac conduction changes, so needs careful monitoring.

Other antidepressants such as mirtazepine and duloxetine are less commonly used.

Antipsychotic medication

Antipsychotic medication is usually used for psychiatric illnesses in which the person is suffering from psychosis. Psychosis can be understood as a loss of contact with reality. People may have hallucinations (hearing voices) or delusions (e.g. believing that they are being followed). Psychosis is most closely associated with schizophrenia, but can also occur in mood disorders.

Doctors also use antipsychotic medication in people with a learning disability to treat challenging behaviour, although there is no evidence to support this use.

Antipsychotic medication can also be used to lessen anxiety, decrease levels of arousal and decrease aggression.

There are two main classes of antipsychotics – the older drugs (known as typical antipsychotics) and the newer ones (known as atypical antipsychotics). There is also a medication called clozapine, which doesn't fall neatly into either group.

Typical antipsychotics

Typical antipsychotics commonly used are: chlorpromazine and haloperidol. These are very effective drugs, but have the potential to cause problematic side-effects. Common side-effects are sedation, dry mouth and weight gain. These drugs can also affect pituitary hormones, causing lactation and changes in menstrual cycle. They tend to cause people to be less fertile. People will commonly develop movement disorders: stiffness, tremor, rabbit-like movements of the mouth. Over long periods of time, people taking these drugs develop tardive dyskinesia. This is a disorder similar to a tic disorder in which people make involuntary movements of the jaw, tongue and fingers. For this reason, these drugs are used less frequently than before and are given with medication (procyclidine) to lessen motor side-effects.

Neuroleptic malignant syndrome is a rare but potentially fatal early side-effect of treatment with typical antipsychotics. The patient develops a high temperature, unstable blood pressure, flushing of the skin and muscle rigidity. This is a medical emergency and requires immediate hospital admission.

Atypical antipsychotics

These are newer antipsychotics, with fewer of the movement side-effects of the typical antipsychotics and less potential to cause neuroleptic malignant syndrome. The ones commonly used are: risperidone, olanzapine, quetiapine, aripiprazole, amisulpiride and asenapine. Although with fewer movement side-effects, these drugs have significant metabolic side-effects, potentially causing weight gain, raised cholesterol and increasing the risk of diabetes. For this reason, regular blood tests and weight measurement are important. They may also affect cardiac conduction, so an annual ECG is a further monitoring requirement. Like the typical antipsychotics, they can cause sedation.

Risperidone in a low dose is used in managing some of the hypersensitivity and hyperarousal experienced by people with autistic spectrum disorders. It has been shown to decrease irritability and repetitive behaviours in this patient group.

Clozapine

Clozapine is an old antipsychotic that works in a similar way to the newer atypical antipsychotic drugs. It is an extremely effective drug for the treatment of schizophrenia but can have potentially fatal side-effects by causing agranulocytosis. For this reason, it is only used after two antipsychotic drugs have been tried without success. It requires very close monitoring and is usually initiated in hospital. Once the person is stable, they continue to require regular monitoring.

49 Antiepileptic drugs

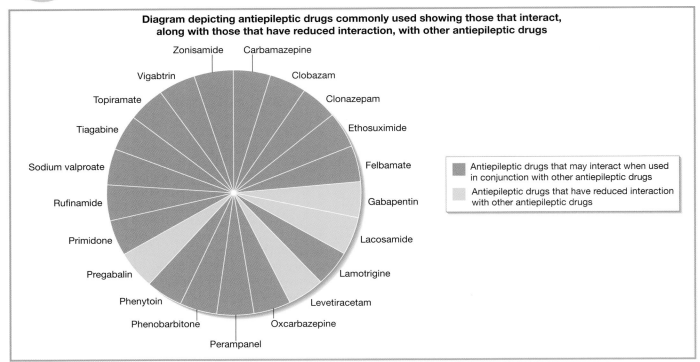

Diagram depicting antiepileptic drugs commonly used showing those that interact, along with those that have reduced interaction, with other antiepileptic drugs

Zonisamide
Carbamazepine
Vigabtrin
Clobazam
Topiramate
Clonazepam
Tiagabine
Ethosuximide
Sodium valproate
Felbamate
Rufinamide
Gabapentin
Primidone
Lacosamide
Pregabalin
Lamotrigine
Phenytoin
Levetiracetam
Phenobarbitone
Oxcarbazepine
Perampanel

Legend:
- Antiepileptic drugs that may interact when used in conjunction with other antiepileptic drugs
- Antiepileptic drugs that have reduced interaction with other antiepileptic drugs

Epilepsy

A seizure is caused by sudden burst of excess electrical activity in the brain causing a temporary disruption in the normal messages passing between brain cells. A person is diagnosed with epilepsy if they have recurring seizures (more than two seizures). Epilepsy seizures are usually divided into generalised and focal seizures.

Many types of epilepsy are referred to as epilepsy syndromes. This means that doctors have recognised that certain clusters of symptoms, signs, patient characteristics and electroencephalogram (EEG detects the brains electrical activity) investigations collectively produce a recognizable pattern. The syndromes notably associated with learning disabilities and epilepsy are Rett's, Landau Kleffner and Lennox-Gastaut syndrome and the seizures are difficult to control.

Why are drugs given for epilepsy?

Medication is taken to prevent epileptic seizures; antiepileptic drug (AED) is the term used for this type of medication in epilepsy. They stop the excessive firing of neurones which causes a seizure.

Most antiepileptic drugs have multiple mechanisms of action on the brain.
• The medication works by stabilising the electrical activities (discharges) in the brain.
• Epilepsy drugs stop or decrease the frequency and intensity of the seizures.

Polypharmacy

Most drugs can be taken safely with all the antiepileptic drugs; however, there are some exceptions. Certain medications may interfere with the antiepileptic drugs therefore it is important to let the doctor know what medication the person is taking. The reason for this is some of the AED drugs interact with , for example, the oral contraceptive pill and other medications such as antidepressants, while antipsychotics lower the seizure threshold.

Side-effects of AEDs

It is essential that people tell their doctor about the other prescribed medication they are receiving. Sometimes interactions may provide an explanation for some side-effects or an increase of seizure frequency.

It is important to monitor a person with learning disabilities when they are prescribed antiepileptic medication, especially as these individuals often have communication problems so are not able to say whether they are experiencing side-effects or problems with their drugs. Therefore they are reliant on their carers being informed, observing and advocating on their behalf to oversee their drug regime and liaising with appropriate health practitioners to address concerns.

• **Allergic hypersensitive (idiosyncratic) side-effects**: These are very rare and happen within one or two weeks of starting the drug. The effects are usually unpredictable and the drug will have to be stopped. The symptoms tend to be a widespread itchy rash.

• **Dose related side-effects**: These side-effects could be linked with the drug being introduced too quickly or by having too much. Most antiepileptic drugs can cause side-effects which include drowsiness, unsteadiness, nausea, blurred or double vision. These effects can be avoided by starting the drug more slowly; they disappear if the dose is reduced.
• **Long-term or chronic side-effects**: These side-effects develop over a number of months or years. They are more common in patients that are on a number of AED drugs and high doses. These effects are often seen in the older drugs, for example phenobarbitone (shoulder joint causing stiffness and pain), phenytoin (gum swelling; slight excess facial hair) rather than the newer drugs

Approaches to prevent side-effects of AEDs

Dose related side-effects may be avoided by the use of sustained or controlled release preparation drugs. The drug (i.e. Tegretol Retard, Epilim Chrono) is released more slowly into the blood reducing the chance of dose related side-effects.

When a person with learning disabilities has co-morbidities (other conditions, e.g. mental health) requiring medication it is preferable to treat the seizure disorder with an antiepileptic drug that has a low interaction potential, for example Levetiracetam or Gabapentin. Refer to the Figure above for the anti-epileptic drugs and potential interactions of these medications.

If a person has epilepsy and takes antiepileptic medication they are exempt from prescription charges for all their prescriptions. They need an exemption certificate which is obtainable from their pharmacy.

Often a person requires a lifelong medication depending on their diagnosis.

The goal for epilepsy treatment is for the best seizure control with the least drug side-effects consistent with optimal quality of life for the individual.

Role of LD nurse

It is recommended that adults who have epilepsy are seen by an epilepsy nurse who they can contact between schedule reviews. Working with the person with learning disabilities and carers there are a number of tasks the nurse will facilitate to improve care:
• A resource for information and advice about epilepsy (ensure the patient /client or carers keep a seizure diary).
• Offering education, counselling and support tailored to individual needs.
• Reducing psychosocial problems in order to improving quality of care.
• Education with patients about their condition (self-management) and to the patient's families/carers/other health professionals, such as ambulance technicians.
• Supporting the doctors – developing guidelines for epilepsy emergency rescue medication, that is buccal midazolam / rectal diazepam.

50 Nurse prescribing

Building a Partnership

1 Listening	2 Communicates
Listens actively to the patient	Helps the patient to interpret information in a way that is meaningful to them

Communication skills, including use of augmentive communication and application of knowledge and experience of how people with a learning disability communicate a range of information including observation of the individual and signs and symptoms of illness	Ability to provide information in an accessible format based upon the communication needs of people with a learning disability

Managing a Shared Consultation

3 Context	4 Knowledge
With the patient defines and agrees the purpose of the consultation	Has up-to-date knowledge of area of practice and wider health services

Nursing assessment, nursing diagnoses, person-centred planning, health action planning	Therapeutic framework, clinical guidelines (i.e. NICE), clinical experience and expertise, clinical governance, pharmacological and prescribing practice guidelines, legislation, evidence-based practice

Sharing a Decision

5 Understanding	6 Exploring	7 Deciding	8 Monitoring
Recognises that the patient is an individual	Discusses illness and treatment options, including no treatment	Decides with the patient the best management strategy	Agrees with the patient what happens next

5	6	7	8
Person-centred legislation, Mental Capacity Act	Knowledge of treatment options, use of personal formulary to inform prescribing practice. Application of Mental Capacity Act and Best Interest Decision Making if individual lacks capacity. Provision of information in accessible format for the individual	Shared care planning, application of Mental Capacity Act and Best Interest Decision Making	Medication review, ongoing monitoring of medical need, clinical management plan to support supplementary prescribing

Learning Disability Nursing at a Glance, First Edition. Edited by Bob Gates, Debra Fearns and Jo Welch. © 2015 John Wiley & Sons, Ltd. Published 2015 by John Wiley & Sons, Ltd.
Companion website: www.ataglanceseries.com/nursing/learningdisability

The role of the learning disability nurse (LDN) as a non-medical prescriber

Non-medical prescribing was initially introduced in 1986. Development of these roles was limited to district nurses and health visitors and specific areas of care. Since 2002 there have been significant changes within policy, opening up non-medical prescribing (NMP) to nurses as supplementary prescribers and the introducing independent prescribing.

NMP is relatively new within the speciality of learning disability nursing. This is not surprising considering the complexity of assessment due to communication difficulties, differential diagnosis, potential of diagnostic overshadowing and the complexity of the drug groups prescribed. People with a learning disability also experience poorer health than the population as a whole. High incidence of health needs increases the potential of polypharmacy, resulting in an increased risk of drug interactions and adverse reactions. Due to these complexities, independent prescribing within learning disability nursing (LDN) is rare with the majority of those qualified to prescribe doing so as supplementary prescribers.

Working with people with a learning disability the NMP must ensure that they are working in partnership with the service user, carers, medical prescriber, pharmacist and the multidisciplinary team to ensure accurate assessment, effective clinical decision making and safe prescribing practice. It is the application of the LDN's specialist knowledge and skills in the health needs of people with a learning disability alongside in-depth pharmacological knowledge and advanced clinical decision making that enables the LDN to prescribe safely.

To undertake NMP the practitioner must have successfully achieved a recordable programme of study through an approved Higher Education Institution (HEI) leading to a registered qualification with the NMC. The nurse must also meet the requirements of the NMC Standards of Proficiency for Nurse and Midwife Prescribers (2006) and work within legislative frameworks including; The Medicines Act 1968 and The Medicinal Products: Prescriptions by Nurses and Others Act 1992. Legislation for medicines management is central to the governance of prescribing practice.

Nurses are accountable practitioners and it is essential that they prescribe within their scope of experience and competency (NMC, 2006). The Figure above provides a framework for NMP for people with a learning disability. This framework emphasises the use of the shared decision-making framework, therapeutic framework and personal drug formulary to inform effective and safe prescribing

practice. The combination of these tools supports the nurse in applying pharmacological and clinical knowledge, clinical skills and clinical decision making to work in partnership with people with a learning disability, family and carers as appropriate. The therapeutic framework supports this and is a tool enabling the NMP to have a clear knowledge base of the clinical health conditions that they are treating. This includes:

- clinical knowledge of the clinical condition;
- medicines used to treat the clinical condition and how they are used;
- pharmacoeconomics (cost benefit of medicines);
- patient and clinical monitoring;
- evidence-based guidelines;
- medicines management;
- NMP role;
- clinical governance;
- integrated approaches to medicines management.

The personal formulary provides a detailed description of the medication that the NMP is likely to prescribe in line with the clinical health conditions they are treating. Within learning disability nursing, NMPs are likely to prescribe antiepileptics and neuroleptics for the treatment of epilepsy, mental illness and emotional distress. The NMP must have advanced knowledge of how drugs interact, adverse drug reactions and contraindications affecting pharmacodynamics and pharmacokinetics of the drugs being prescribed.

Due to the risk of polypharmacy in this population group it is recommended that the principles of prescribing for the elderly outlined within the British National Formulary (BNF) are followed. The BNF recommend simplifying drug regimes, reduced dose, regular medication review, clear advice and education. The reason for these principles to be applied is that as a result of having a learning disability and abnormalities of the brain, people with a learning disability can experience altered sensitivities to drugs, changed effects of drugs and there can be difficulties in determining the optimum dose.

Summary

- NMP is a relatively new role for learning disability nurses.
- LD nurses need to undertake a recordable programme of study at an approved university and then register this qualification with the NMC.
- Legislation for medicines management is central to the governance of prescribing practice.

Drug calculations

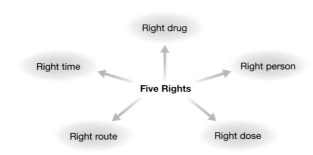

Five Rights

- Right drug
- Right time
- Right person
- Right route
- Right dose

Common volumes of measurement used within medicines management

Unit of Measurement	Unit	Abbreviated to	Equivalent to
Units of Volume	1 litre	l	1000 ml
Units of Mass	1 kilogram	kg	1000 g
	1 gram	g	1000 mg
	1 milligram	mg	1000 microgram
	1 microgram	Microgram (not abbreviated)	
Units of Amount	1 mole	mol	1000 millimole
	1 millimole	mmol	

DRUG NAME ◄

Indications details of clinical uses

Cautions details of precautions required and also any monitoring required
Counselling Verbal explanation to the patient of specific details of the drug treatment (e.g. posture when taking a medicine)

Contra-indications circumstances when a drug should be avoided

Hepatic impairment advice on the use of a drug in hepatic impairment

Renal impairment advice on the use of a drug in renal impairment

Pregnancy advice on the use of a drug during pregnancy

Breast-feeding advice on the use of a drug during breast-feeding

Side-effects very common (greater than 1 in 10) and common (1 in 100 to 1 in 10); *less commonly* (1 in 1000 to 1 in 100); *rarely* (1 in 10 000 to 1 in 1000); *very rarely* (less than 1 in 10 000); also reported, frequency not known

Dose
- Dose and frequency of administration (max. dose); CHILD and ELDERLY details of dose for specific age group
- By alternative route, dose and frequency

¹Approved Name (Non-proprietary) (PoM) ◄
Pharmaceutical form, sugar-free, active ingredient mg/mL, net price, pack size = basic NHS price. Label: (as in Appendix 3)
1. Exceptions to the prescribing status are indicated by a note or footnote.

Proprietary Name (Manufacturer) (PoM) (NHS) ◄
Pharmaceutical form, colour, coating, active ingredient and amount in dosage form, net price, pack size = basic NHS price. Label: (as in Appendix 3)
Excipients include clinically important excipients
Electrolytes clinically significant quantities of electrolytes
Note Specific notes about the product e.g. handling

Preparations
Preparations are included under a non-proprietary title, if they are marketed under such a title, if they are not otherwise prescribable under the NHS, or if they may be prepared extemporaneously.

Drugs
Drugs appear under pharmacopoeial or other non-proprietary titles. When there is an *appropriate current monograph* (Human Medicines Regulations 2012) preference is given to a name at the head of that monograph; otherwise a British Approved Name (BAN), if available, is used.

The symbol ◢ is used to denote those preparations that are considered by the Joint Formulary Committee to be less suitable for prescribing. Although such preparations may not be considered as drugs of first choice, their use may be justifiable in certain circumstances.

Prescription-only medicines (PoM)
This symbol has been placed against those preparations that are available only on a prescription issued by an appropriate practitioner. For more detailed information see *Medicines, Ethics and Practice*, London, Pharmaceutical Press (always consult latest edition).

The symbols (CD2) (CD3) (CD4-1) (CD4-2) indicate that the preparations are subject to the prescription requirements of the Misuse of Drugs Act. For regulations governing prescriptions for such preparations see Controlled Drugs and Drug Dependence.

Preparations not available for NHS prescription (NHS)
This symbol has been placed against those preparations included in the BNF that are not prescribable under the NHS. Those prescribable only for specific disorders have a footnote specifying the condition(s) for which the preparation remains available. Some preparations which are not *prescribable* by brand name under the NHS may nevertheless be *dispensed* using the brand name providing that the prescription shows an appropriate non-proprietary name.

Prices
Prices have been calculated from the basic cost used in pricing NHS prescriptions, see also Prices in the BNF for details.

Learning Disability Nursing at a Glance, First Edition. Edited by Bob Gates, Debra Fearns and Jo Welch. © 2015 John Wiley & Sons, Ltd. Published 2015 by John Wiley & Sons, Ltd.
Companion website: www.ataglanceseries.com/nursing/learningdisability

Introduction

This chapter will provide an overview of the learning disability nurse's role in administration of medication, the standards and frameworks governing practice and basic drug calculation formula to support safe medication administration practice.

Incidents related to medicines management account for the third largest cause of incidents reported to the National Patient Safety Agency (NPSA). Although the large majority of these incidents do not result in significant harm to individuals, the most serious incidents can result in death. The largest proportion of errors is during administration of medication. Although a range of professionals are involved in medicines management, the nurse is the last line of protection in ensuring that patients are administered medication correctly and safely. Therefore nurses must be competent in knowledge of medication, medicines management and safety, clinical decision making and drug calculations.

To support nurses in safe medicines management, learning disability nurses must ensure they are competent in and working within the NMC Standards for Medicines Management (2010). This includes knowledge of common drug groups prescribed for people with a learning disability and clinical assessment and decision making skills based upon the presenting needs of the individual.

In administering any medication it is essential for the nurse to ensure that they are administering the correct medication to the correct person, at the correct dose, through the correct route, at the correct time. They must also ensure knowledge of the therapeutic use of the drug, therapeutic dose range, precautions, contraindications and side-effects as well as checking the prescription, drug label and expiry date. Safe administration of medication is not merely a task where the nurse follows the guidance of a prescription; it is a technical clinical role where the nurse must demonstrate clinical judgements and decision making in order to ensure correct and safe administration.

Drug calculations

In order to undertake drug calculations, nurses must have basic mathematical skills including; multiplication, division, fractions, decimals, percentages, units of measurement and concentrations. The most common units of measurement used within medicines management are mass and volume.

Tablets and capsules

The most common form of medication is tablets and capsules. In order to undertake a drug calculation the nurse must check the dose (also referred to as strength required) and route of administration on the prescription/drug chart. They must also check the drug packaging for the drug name and the drug strength (also referred to as stock strength). This information provides the nurse with the necessary information to calculate the required dose. This is done by dividing the strength required by the stock strength.

For example, if Patient A is prescribed 400 mg Carbamazepine and the drug label was Carbamazepine ® 100 mg tablets the dose calculation would be:

$$\frac{\text{Strength required}\left(400\,\text{mg}\right)}{\text{Stock strength}\left(100\,\text{mg}\right)} = \text{Volume required}\left(4\,\text{tablets}\right)$$

Liquid and oral Solutions

Liquid medications are commonly prescribed for people with a learning disability due to swallowing difficulties. With liquid medication the dose is calculated in millilitres (ml). The nurse must calculate the amount of medication required based upon the strength required, divided by the stock strength and multiplied by the volume of stock solution. For example if patient B is prescribed Fluoxetine 60 mg in liquid form and the drug label is Fluoxetine ® 20 mg in 5 ml the dose calculation would be:

$$\frac{\text{Strength required}\left(60\,\text{mg}\right)}{\text{Stock strength}\left(20\,\text{mg}\right)} \times \text{Volume of stock solution}\left(5\,\text{ml}\right)$$
$$= \text{Volume required (15 ml)}$$

Injections

The largest proportion of incidents reported to the NPSA resulting in death or severe harm were related to injectable medicines. It is essential that the administering nurse has knowledge of the medication being administered, the route (intramuscular/intravenous) and the corresponding therapeutic dose range. Injectable medication comes in different strengths and various volumes, careful attention must be paid to these to ensure accurate drug calculation. To calculate the volume required the formula below can be used. This formula is illustrated with the following example: Patient C is prescribed Aripiprazole 9.75 mg and the drug label is Aripiprazole 7.5 mg/ml. To calculate the volume of dose required the nurse must multiply the strength required by the volume of stock solution. This must then be divided by the stock strength in order to ascertain the correct volume required to be administered.

$$\frac{\text{Strength required}\left(9.75\,\text{mg}\right) \times \text{Volume of stock solution}\left(1\,\text{ml}\right)}{\text{Stock strength}\left(7.5\,\text{mg}\right)}$$
$$= \text{Volume required}\left(1.3\,\text{ml}\right)$$

Conversions

If the unit of measurement for the prescribed dose and the information on the drug label are different, it is advised that the larger unit of measurement is converted to the smaller unit of measurement to avoid risk of error. For example if Patient A is prescribed 1 g Paracetamol and the drug label is:

PARACETAMOL	500 mg tablets

The nurse must convert g to mg. This is done by multiplying by 1000. The calculation would be: 1 x 1000 = 1000 mg. The volume required would then be calculated using the appropriate drug calculation formula above.

Summary
• Drug administration is complex. All nurses must ensure that they are competent in all aspects of medicines management, including drug calculations, and are working within the NMC guidelines and local policies and procedures.

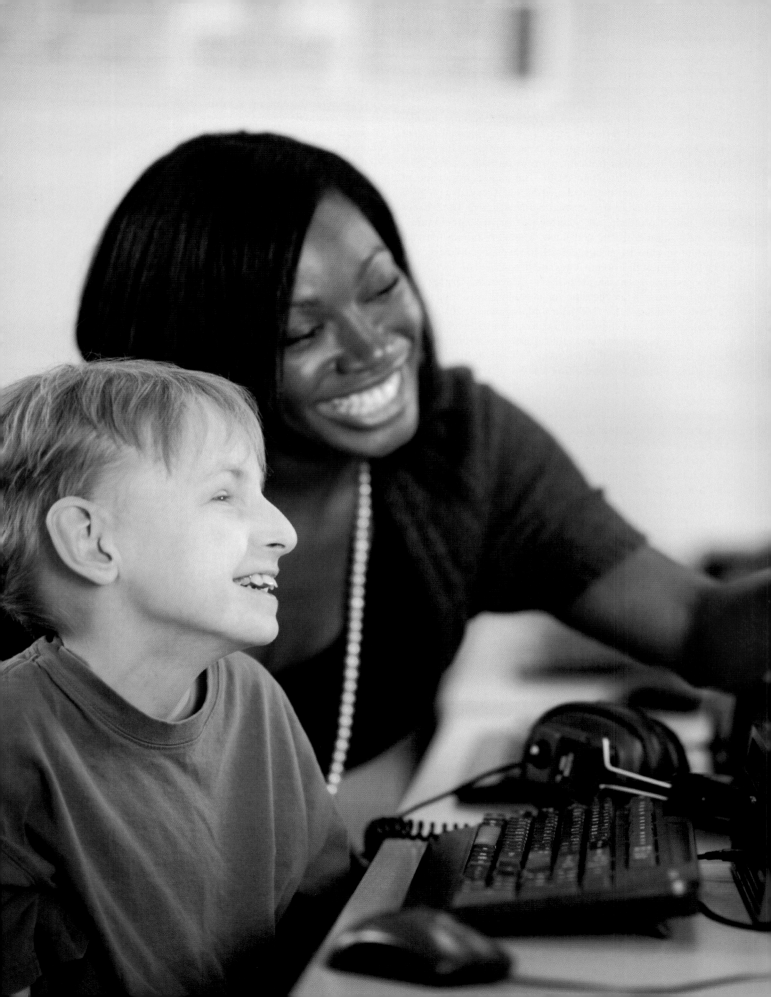

The learning disability nurse

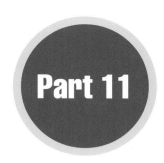

Part 11

Chapters

52 **The community learning disability nurse** 122
53 **Healthcare facilitators** 124
54 **The health liaison nurse** 126
55 **The assessment and treatment learning disability nurse** 128
56 **The prison nurse** 130

Don't forget to visit the companion website for this book at **www.ataglanceseries.com/nursing/learningdisability** to do some practice cases on these topics.

52 The community learning disability nurse

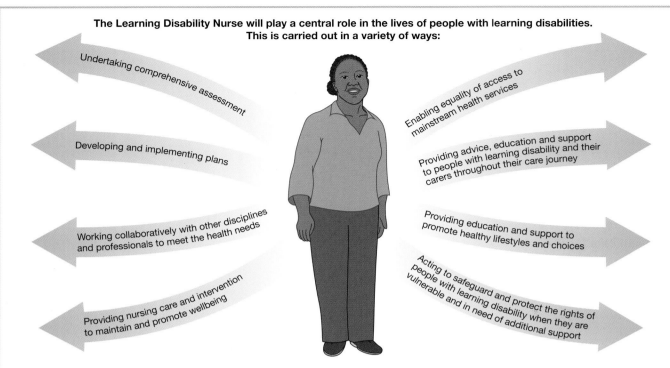

The Learning Disability Nurse will play a central role in the lives of people with learning disabilities. This is carried out in a variety of ways:

Undertaking comprehensive assessment

Developing and implementing plans

Working collaboratively with other disciplines and professionals to meet the health needs

Providing nursing care and intervention to maintain and promote wellbeing

Enabling equality of access to mainstream health services

Providing advice, education and support to people with learning disability and their carers throughout their care journey

Providing education and support to promote healthy lifestyles and choices

Acting to safeguard and protect the rights of people with learning disability when they are vulnerable and in need of additional support

Skills and qualities of the community learning disability nurse

Communication

Learning disability nurses have highly tuned communication skills. They listen and really hear what the person is communicating, they are highly skilled interpreters of body language and behaviours and of course of the spoken word.

Empathy

Learning disability nurses respect the individual they are supporting, they listen, and because they have the other skills and qualities listed in this box, they have the ability to understand and share the feelings of the individual. If this is missing then how can the nurse claim to be person-centred?

Innovation/creativity

Learning disability nurses 'think outside of the box'. They can assess a situation and find creative and innovative solutions. Learning disability nurses are not traditionally task-orientated and so have much more freedom to be creative.

Commitment

Learning disability nurses pride themselves on the fact that they 'walk the journey' with the individual and their family/carers. In partnership they agree the plan of action and they walk beside the individual until the outcome is met.

Holistic/person-centred approach

Learning disability nurses have the ability to look at the individual as a whole person and recognise how all the other aspects of an individual's life impact on their health. They support the individual as a partner in order to reach the health goal. The individual remains at the heart of their care.

Patience

Learning disability nurses recognise that the progress in reaching the desired health outcome may be slow and the individual may need a lot of prompting for small steps forward. Sometimes the plan doesn't work and the process must start over. The nurse never loses their focus in achieving the shared goal.

Advocate

Learning disability nurses have core skills, particularly the ability to advocate. Historically, people with learning disabilities have been a marginalised group; learning disability nurses have been key to publicly supporting and advocating for the rights of the individual – equity in accessing mainstream health services being an example.

(Learning from the Past – Setting Out the Future: Developing Learning Disability Nursing in the United Kingdom. An RCN Position Statement on the Role of the LD Nurse. January 2011.)

Fact: *There are approximately 1.5 million people in Britain living with learning disabilities, this number is likely to increase by 14% between 2001 and 2021* (Emerson & Hatton, 2008).

Background

With the closure of long-stay hospitals for people with learning disabilities and the shift in political and social agendas, and the advancement in medical science, people with learning disabilities are now living longer and more fulfilled lives.

Learning disability nursing has always played an important role in the healthcare of people with learning disabilities and so you would expect the growth of learning disability nursing as a discipline to be increasing with the rising population. However, this is not the case, the number of learning disability nurses is decreasing as many near retirement and others transfer their skills and seek employment in independent sectors.

The role of the learning disability nurse

A key characteristic of the role of the community LD nurse is the ability to keep the person with learning disability at the very centre of their care. They are able to interpret the sometimes over complicated and jargonistic world and help it make sense to the individual, whether this is in adapting written information into easy read information or getting to the root of why somebody's behaviour is challenging, the examples could be endless. They take the complicated and deconstruct it into manageable chunks and then reconstruct it again in a meaningful way. They have a broad knowledge, not just of their role but the role of other professionals and services and are able to ensure that the individual and their families receive the appropriate service to meet their specific needs at a time when it is needed.

The role of the community LD nurse is evolving with an emphasis much more on health facilitation and specialist roles within community learning disability teams.

The guidance set out in Department of Health Good Practice in Learning Disability Nursing (2007) endorses the expectation in Valuing People (DoH, 2001) that learning disability nurses will engage in a range of activities additional to a direct clinical role. The range of activities includes:

- Health promotion – working closely with the local health promotion team.
- Health facilitation – working with primary care teams, community health professionals and staff delivering secondary healthcare.
- Teaching – to enable a wide range of staff, including those who work in social services and the independent sector, to become more familiar with how to support people with learning disabilities to have their health needs met.
- Service development – contributing their knowledge of health issues to planning processes.

Learning disability nurses are unique in that they are able to 'walk the journey' with the individual, they can help the individual and their carers/family members to 'unlock the doors' along the journey to enable equity of healthcare services, which historically have been closed.

The community LD nurse has a 'virtual back pack' which they take with them on the journey, this includes their skills, qualities and experience all combined into an essential toolkit, they may not need all the elements in the toolkit all the time but they know they are always there in their back pack when they are needed.

Community Learning Disability Nurses have developed into highly specialised nurses over recent years but they rarely lose their background (Gates, 2009).

Summary

- The population of people with learning disabilities is increasing.
- The number of learning disability nurses is decreasing.
- The core skills and qualities of community learning disability nurses are: communication, empathy, innovation/creativity, commitment, holistic/person-centred care, patience, advocating.
- Learning disability nurses work in a creative, person-centred manner to support the individual, sometimes long term, to reach their health potential.
- The role of the community learning disability nurse is evolving, with more focus on health facilitation and improving the access to mainstream services.
- The role of the community learning disability nurse has become more specialised but they rarely lose their background.

53 Healthcare facilitators

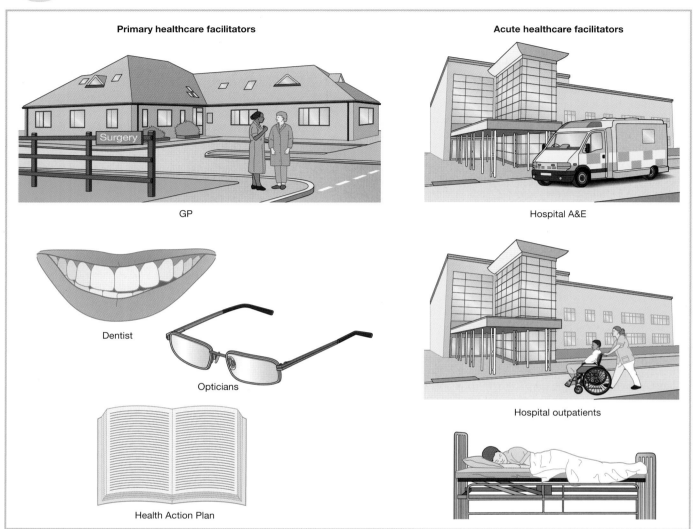

Primary healthcare facilitators

GP

Dentist

Opticians

Health Action Plan

Acute healthcare facilitators

Hospital A&E

Hospital outpatients

Introduction

South Essex Partnership University NHS Foundation Trust is committed to supporting people who have a learning disability and to providing a model of community-based health facilitation to work alongside existing adult community learning disability teams within the local authorities and with colleagues in primary care and the two acute hospitals in Bedfordshire and Luton.

The nurse-led service which is mirrored in many areas across the UK, provides support for people who have a learning disability to access primary, secondary, tertiary and acute healthcare services that are fit for purpose, effective and safe for people who have a learning disability, including access to the National Health Screening Programmes.

Essentially this service is 'to enable people with Learning Disabilities to access health services designed around their individual needs, with fast and convenient care delivered to a consistently high standard, and with additional support where necessary'

(Valuing People, 2001). Health facilitators work alongside people who have a learning disability, their family and carers as well as other healthcare providers to ensure that person-centred care is delivered.

Primary healthcare facilitators

In Bedfordshire and Luton the primary health facilitators are based within the three local authority community teams for people who have a learning disability. There is one nurse specialist and one clinical support worker to cover each area. The clinical support worker will assist the nurse specialist.

The nurse specialists will:
• Make contact with healthcare providers in their area including practice managers, GPs, district nurses, dentists, opticians and other specialist services.
• Ensure that mainstream services are able to provide healthcare services to people who have a learning disability that are safe,

effective and fit for purpose through the use of reasonable adjustments (Equality Act, 2010), and provide specialist training where appropriate.

• Promote the importance and use of Health Action Plans to maintain health and wellbeing.

• Support GPs to engage with the Directed Enhanced Services for People with Learning Disabilities (DES 2008–2013) and ensure that annual health checks are offered and delivered to people who have a learning disability.

• Support people who have a learning disability to access physical healthcare appointments.

• Ensure that people who have a learning disability understand the outcomes of their healthcare appointments.

• Support engagement in Health Promotion Activities with people who have a learning disability and their carers.

• Aim to reduce inappropriate admissions to acute hospital by providing support to access primary care for early detection of illness.

• Provide support to the person who has a learning disability, their carers and hospital staff by working collaboratively with the liaison nurses at Bedford Hospital and the Luton and Dunstable Hospital.

Acute healthcare facilitators

In Bedfordshire and Luton there are two acute hospitals. At each hospital there is one lead learning disability liaison nurse and one junior learning disability liaison nurse.

The hospital learning disability liaison nurses will:

• Work collaboratively with the primary health facilitators to plan admission and discharge into and out of acute care.

• Develop identification systems (flagging) and pathways to ensure easy access to acute healthcare.

• Ensure that mainstream services are able to provide healthcare services to people who have a learning disability that are safe, effective and fit for purpose through the use of reasonable adjustments (Equality Act, 2010), and provide specialist training where appropriate.

• Support people who have a learning disability to access physical healthcare appointments.

• Ensure that people who have a learning disability understand the outcomes of their healthcare appointments or admissions.

• Promote a safe and effective discharge from acute care back into the community by working with the person who has a learning disability, their family and carers and other health and or social care professionals to ensure their needs are met.

54 The health liaison nurse

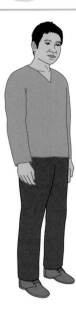

The Health Facilitator

Primary role: to ensure that people with learning disabilities gain access to better healthcare

Strategic organisational work:
- networking and identifying local health resources and health services
- developing relationships with healthcare providers (e.g. dentists/podiatrists/tissue viability teams/continence services)
- developing and contributing towards care pathways (e.g. screening services/maternity)
- working with GP practices to refine their learning disability databases
- delivery of the DES (Direct Enhanced Service) to ensure that people with learning disabilities receive annual health checks

Individual interventions:
- to address the barriers and obstacles that can prevent good access to healthcare

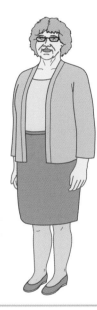

The Hospital Liaison Nurse

Primary role: to promote effective communication, better planning and discharge, better compliance to treatment and treatment options, and improved staff understanding of learning disability issues

Provides:
- support and advice on attending outpatient appointments
- planning elective surgery
- support to patients in emergencies
- training to hospital staff
- advice on reasonable adjustments
- knowledge about Mental Capacity Act, Safeguarding, Deprivation of Liberty issues
- support and advice on discharge planning

Learning Disability Nursing at a Glance, First Edition. Edited by Bob Gates, Debra Fearns and Jo Welch. © 2015 John Wiley & Sons, Ltd. Published 2015 by John Wiley & Sons, Ltd.
Companion website: www.ataglanceseries.com/nursing/learningdisability

Health liaison nurse

Health liaison is a term that can be open to interpretation. There are many roles within specialist learning disability services that will liaise with other services to improve both health and social care services for people with a learning disability. However, in more recent years there are two distinctive roles that have developed to improve not only access to better health services for individuals, but to work within those services, thereby improving communications and ultimately pathways of care. These roles are the health facilitator and the hospital liaison nurse.

The role of the health facilitator was developed in response to the Valuing People white paper (DoH, 2001). The brief for this role was to support people with a learning disability to access health services. The term 'health facilitator' can be ambiguous as the role does not have to be performed solely by a health professional – it can also be undertaken by a family member, an advocate or social care staff. The Department of Health recommends partnership working between primary care and specialist learning disability services so there are improved health outcomes.

Everyone has a role in facilitating the health needs for people with learning disabilities, but there is clear evidence that suggests that learning disability nurses are ideally placed in being at the forefront in reducing the barriers that exist for people with learning disabilities.

Many learning disability trusts have seen the introduction of the new role of health facilitators and hospital liaison nurses; these are primarily nurses with a learning disability background who play a key role in utilising their knowledge, skills and experience in addressing some of the barriers in healthcare for people with learning disabilities.

As described in the Health Action Planning and Health Facilitation for People with Learning Disabilities; Good Practice Guide (DoH, 2009) the primary role of the health facilitator is to ensure that people with learning disabilities get better healthcare.

The work of the health facilitator is best described as being on two levels. First is the strategic organisational work which includes: networking and identifying local health resources and health services, developing relationships with healthcare providers (for example- dentists/podiatrists/tissue viability teams/continence services), developing and contributing towards care pathways (for example- screening services/maternity), working with GP practices to refine their learning disability databases and the delivery of the DES (Direct Enhanced Service) to ensure that people with learning disabilities receive their annual health checks.

Second are the individual interventions in addressing the barriers and obstacles that prevent good access to healthcare. An example of this is best demonstrated in the following scenario.

A gentleman with moderate learning disabilities was referred to the local learning disability team. He had type 2 diabetes and he required his annual diabetic health check. All the usual diabetic routine checks had been implemented effectively but he found having a blood test really difficult and anxiety provoking. The health facilitator discussed this prior to his appointment with his carer, GP and practice nurse and agreed that in his best interests to go ahead with the blood tests as this had not be achieved for four years and currently it appeared that his sugar levels were not within the normal safe range. A plan was made and agreed which included a quiet time and longer appointment in the GP surgery, familiar practice nurse and carer support and the use of distraction techniques.

The nurse was successful in taking bloods which confirmed that the gentlemen's diabetic medication needed adjusting. A referral to the specialist diabetic nurse was also prompted at the request of the health facilitator for some carer training on the management of his diabetes and the promotion of a healthier lifestyle. The feedback from the practice nurse included that she would feel more confident in working with people with a learning disability in the future and will adopt similar approaches with regards to the use of reasonable adjustments.

A number of reports (DoH, 2008; Mencap, 2012; RCN, 2010), highlight the communication difficulties between service users, their carers' and hospital staff which have resulted in poor quality hospital care and in some cases deaths. As a result, in more recent years we have seen the development of the hospital (or acute) liaison nurse for people with a learning disability.

The work of the hospital liaison nurse is as equally a challenging role as the health facilitator: 26% of people with learning disability will access hospitals as opposed to 14% of the general population; this clearly identifies challenges for acute services in providing equitable services for people with learning disabilities.

The hospital liaison nurses are based within an acute hospital setting and provide a range of services within the hospital for people with learning disabilities. The hospital liaison nurse can be part of the whole patients journey which can include: support and advice on attending outpatients appointments, planning elective surgery, support to patients in emergencies, training to hospital staff, advice on reasonable adjustments, Mental Capacity Act, Safeguarding, Deprivation of Liberty issues and support and advice on discharge planning.

The benefits of this role include: the ability to promote effective communication, better planning and discharge, better compliance with treatment and treatment options and improved staff understanding of learning disability issues.

Summary

- Acts as a facilitator to help people with learning disabilities access services.
- Works strategically with local health resources and health services.
- Provides direct interventions to support people with learning disabilities when accessing services.
- Hospital liaison nurses' promote effective communication, better planning and discharge, better compliance with treatment and treatment options.

The assessment and treatment learning disability nurse

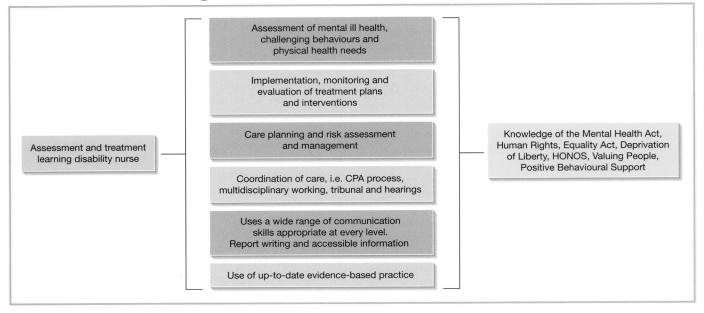

Assessment and treatment learning disability nurse

Assessment of mental ill health, challenging behaviours and physical health needs

Implementation, monitoring and evaluation of treatment plans and interventions

Care planning and risk assessment and management

Coordination of care, i.e. CPA process, multidisciplinary working, tribunal and hearings

Uses a wide range of communication skills appropriate at every level. Report writing and accessible information

Use of up-to-date evidence-based practice

Knowledge of the Mental Health Act, Human Rights, Equality Act, Deprivation of Liberty, HONOS, Valuing People, Positive Behavioural Support

Assessment and treatment A&T learning disability (LD) nurses work within a multidisciplinary team to provide a holistic care package for people with a learning disability presenting with severe challenging/offending behaviours, mental ill health difficulties and other complex health issues. This is usually within an inpatient assessment and treatment unit/hospital providing specialist services for people with a learning disability. They are the front-line staff in services designed to meet the needs of service users who are unable to use general services due to their vulnerability or the complexity of their needs. Specialist services are temporary services aimed to provide specialist support at the point of acute need.

A&T LD nurses engage with people with a learning disability and actively work with them and their carers to provide appropriate healthcare. The nurses are responsible for promoting and maintaining the health and wellbeing of service users, in collaboration with a multidisciplinary/clinical team with specialist learning disability expertise, and in partnership with carers and family. As such the assessment and treatment nurse should possess good communication and interpersonal skills, and be able to engage service users in their care and all the relevant professionals, contributing to the Care Programme Approach (CPA).

A&T nurses help to develop care packages with individuals, agreeing outcomes and objectives where possible. They are also instrumental in ensuring the information is in an accessible format for the service user to understand. They are able to observe, report and record changes in the service users physical, mental health and behaviour and have a good understanding of the Mental Health Act and positive behavioural support interventions. They should maintain a working knowledge of legislation, policy and guidance pertaining to mental health, challenging behaviour and learning disabilities to provide the best possible and evidence based care.

Training of unqualified staff and mentoring student nurses is also an essential part of the role of the nurse.

Assessment

The assessment process involved the compilation of information using specialist knowledge and skills in identifying and documenting a person's level of functioning, the current behaviours and mental health state and the general needs of a person. Nurses are responsible for using evidence-based assessment tools in order to, as accurately as possible, assess and monitor mental health presentations and communicate these effectively to the clinical/multidisciplinary team. The nurses work closely with the service user and support workers/carers in compiling a complete assessment of the area of need. This focusses on the development of a therapeutic relationship based on trust and respecting a service users' personal integrity regardless of their challenging behaviour, history or mental health state. The nurse works in a non-judgemental way for the purpose of cultivating a therapeutic environment where service users can express their thoughts and feelings safely, this being the key to a better understanding of their problems and needs.

A&T LD nurses recognize the importance of meaningful activity and access to the locality, in supporting and maintaining good health and wellbeing. There is a focus on engaging individuals and helping to, for example, reduce boredom which has been linked to some challenging behaviours. The aim is for inclusion and participation in society and local activities, with a focus to discharge individuals to local services within a reasonable time frame.

Treatment

A&T LD nurses are also responsible for the skillful implementation of treatment programmes agreed by the clinical team, carers and service user. This includes the application of evidence-based nursing models in assessment, planning, implementation and evaluation. The treatment package is holistic in its approach to both mental health and physical health and takes into account the severity of a person's learning disability.

This is often a complex process involving the monitoring of the effects of medication and/or behaviour treatment plans. The process of treatment is also reflective and seeks to examine why behaviours occur and their function. Risk assessment and management strategies are also in line with trust and local policies, and ensure the safe delivery of care.

The LD nurse also considers the environment, resources and their impact on planning individualised approaches. Constant monitoring and evaluation of treatment plans and shaping and/or adapting intervention strategies to suit individual needs is required.

It is generally recognised that people with a learning disability in the criminal justice system are more likely to re-offend due to a lack of understanding of their needs and insufficient support in general prison services, and would benefit greatly from inpatient services where they can access specialist nursing staff and treatment interventions.

Treatment plans and interventions take a holistic approach to the health and care of people in promoting physical and emotional comfort. This also includes the effective process of transition from hospital, inpatient settings into the community and more independent living. Discharge planning is an integral part of the care and treatment that people receive.

Communication

A&T nurses use a wide range of communication tools as the service user communication is varied and dependent on the level of learning disability and acuteness of mental ill health where appropriate. This ranges from the use of Makaton, objects of reference, checking understanding and the use of short phrases, among others.

Nurses should be able to anticipate service user needs, particularly for those who have difficulty in expressing these, for example, hunger, thirst, toilet use, and be able to establish a routine early after admission in order to reduce anxieties. The nurse therefore possesses a unique set of skills to ensure the safety of the unit/hospital and the management of behaviours.

56 The prison nurse

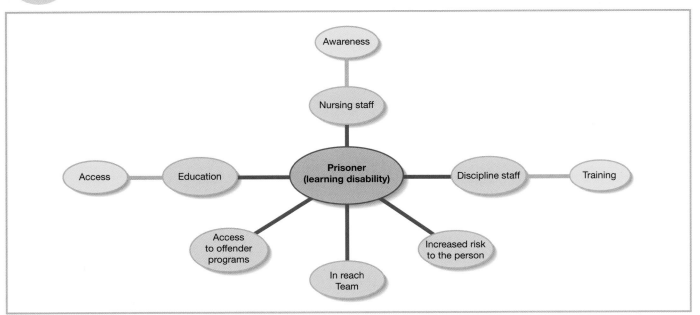

The role of the prison nurse

Learning disability within the criminal justice system is always a complex issue for all concerned. It is hoped that all learning disability offenders will be filtered through to more suitable units than the mainstream prison environment.

There are, however, times when offenders with an LD will be incarcerated. The learning disability may have gone unnoticed/undiagnosed due to:

- Poor/inadequate/absent parenting skills.
- Poor education/non-attendance at school.
- Non-engagement with outside agencies.

The role of the prison nurse is to be able to engage with the LD prisoner, and also involve all of the resources/agencies inside and outside the prison to enable a safe and humane incarceration period. Many aspects of daily life can prove confusing and upsetting for an LD prisoner. There is also a stigma attached to admitting having an LD, such as being seen as vulnerable, potential for being bullied or coerced into doing things for others, labels of MAD, FRAGGLE, and THICK used to be commonplace.

The following is a quote from a female prisoner with learning disabilities in 'Prisoners voices' (Talbot, 2008).

When I first came in I was petrified. The first one and a half years were really bad; I tried to commit suicide three times.

There are aspects of prison life which the LD prisoner will find difficult to deal with and he/she needs a thorough assessment to provide care staff with enough information and education to deal with this prisoner. Daily living issues are of particular importance.

The quotes below are LD prisoners' views on aspects of daily living.

Form filling:

Everything is written for a very educated person and the words are very long. It's really a humiliation if you have to ask someone.

(Talbot, 2008)

Ordering food from wing meal sheets:

I eat the same thing every time; I manage by copying from the previous form.

(Talbot, 2008)

Several reports have been published recently which have identified that the needs of prisoners with a possible or diagnosed learning disability are not being met within the current system.

- The prevalence of individuals with LD in the criminal justice system ranges from 1–10% (Loukes, 2007).

- High risk of recidivism due to unidentified needs, lack of support by services, limited insight into the challenges of working with this group.
- The Bradley Report (2009) highlights the need for better services for offenders with learning disabilities in the criminal justice system.
- The Prison Reform Trust in the report No-one Knows (2007) and Valuing People (2001) recommended key objectives including the monitoring of offenders with LD in custody.
- More often than not, no systematic screening of learning disabilities takes place, nor is information available (Loukes, 2007).

There is a screening tool that has now been developed for nursing staff to enable them to carry out an initial assessment when staff within the prison raise concerns about a prisoner. Reception health screening would often identify if further investigation is required, for example the response from prisoner when asked certain questions.

Taking things forward

Historically, very little has been put in place to deal with this type of prisoner, but things are changing. Much more emphasis is being placed on care and welfare of prisoners with a learning disability. Stronger ties with outside agencies have enabled more structured formal assessments to take place.

Learning disability can have a big impact on efforts that are made to reduce reoffending. Loucks (2007) identifies that:

This group of offenders:

- *are at risk of re-offending because of unidentified needs and consequent lack of support and services*
- *are unlikely to benefit from conventional programmes designed to address offending behaviour*
- *are targeted by other prisoners when in custody*
- *present numerous difficulties for the staff who work with them, especially when these staff often lack specialist training or are unfamiliar with the challenges of working with this group of people.*

The role of the prison nurse will evolve to meet prisoner demand for advocates, educators and informers. We, as nursing staff, are in a unique position in that we can educate and improve the lives of the prisoners in our care.

Being in prison is a frightening experience even for the hardest criminals, imagine how scary it is if you don't know or understand what is going either.

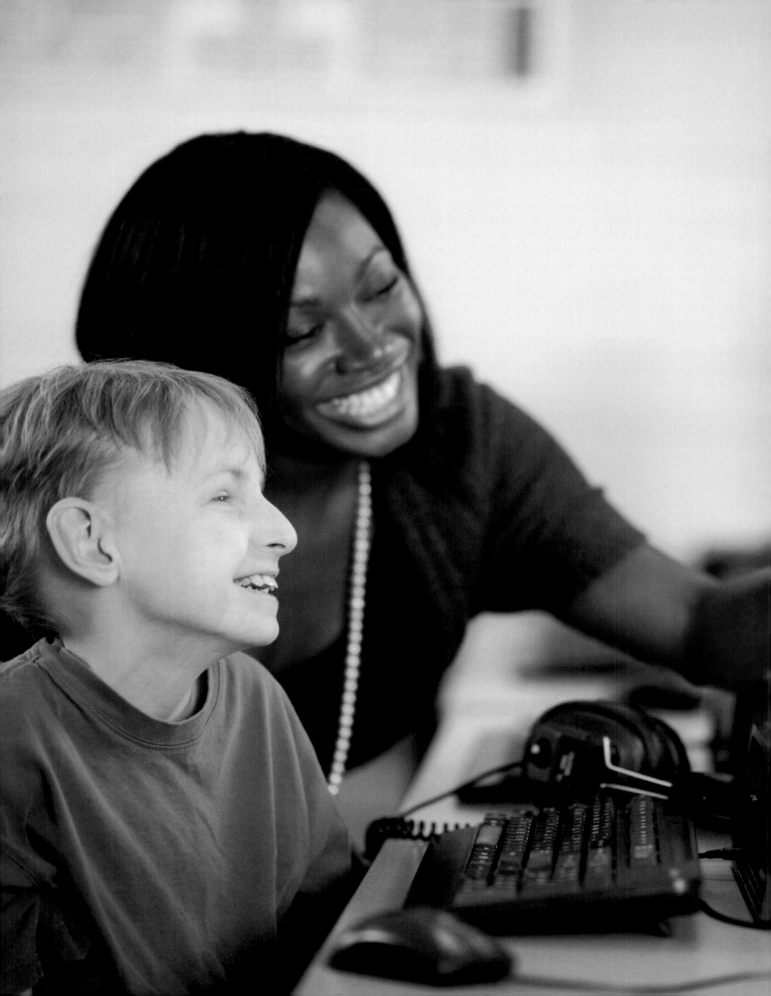

Inclusion

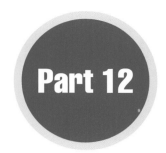

Part 12

Chapters

57 **Person centred planning** 134
58 **Employment** 136
59 **Housing and leisure** 138
60 **Ethnic minorities and learning disability** 140
61 **Parents with a learning disability** 142
62 **Family perspectives** 144
63 **A service user's perspective** 146
64 **Advocacy** 148
65 **Health passports** 150
66 **Hate crime** 151
67 **Sex and individuals with a learning disability** 152
68 **Spirituality** 154
69 **The twenty-first century: Networking for success** 155

Don't forget to visit the companion website for this book at www.ataglanceseries.com/nursing/learningdisability to do some practice cases on these topics.

57 # Person centred planning

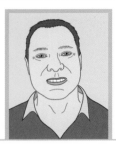

John is in his 40s.
He has severe epilepsy

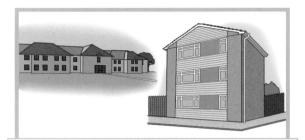

He lived in large residential centres for 20 years up until a few years ago when he moved to a 'shared lives scheme'

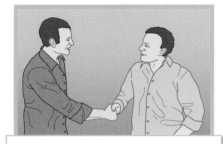

John has a brother who he sees regularly

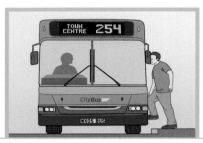

His plan included thinking about:
- keeping safe and healthy
- managing and understanding his epilepsy
- cooking
- gym
- dealing with cold calling

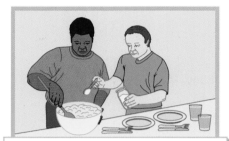

- meals with his shared life family
- bed monitor
- managing his medication
- appointments with GPs and epilepsy nurse
- SOS bracelet

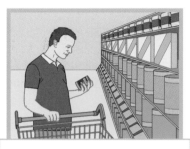

- health action plan
- travel training
- mobile phone
- visit to bank; managing finances
- managing the internet

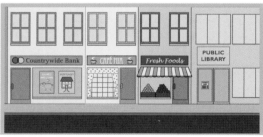

Social/activities/interests

Volunteer jobs – country market and shop; local gym twice a week, volunteer for RSPB, library, planning activity on whiteboard. Watercolour course Wednesday evenings, planning a holiday, using direct funding

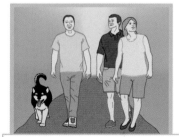

Family

Seeing brother; part of shared lives – family meals, taking dog for a walk – dog jumping on bed in the morning to wake John up

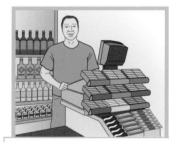

Aims

Work experience and paid work – volunteer on project about quality checking; peer listening, talked about life at university to student social workers

Learning Disability Nursing at a Glance, First Edition. Edited by Bob Gates, Debra Fearns and Jo Welch. © 2015 John Wiley & Sons, Ltd. Published 2015 by John Wiley & Sons, Ltd.
Companion website: www.ataglanceseries.com/nursing/learningdisability

Introduction

Person-centred planning considers how an individual wants to live and what needs to be done to achieve this. There is not one set way of person-centred planning, but rather a collection of tools and approaches based on the values of inclusion.

Person-centred planning is used to plan *with* a person – not *for* them. It should build the person's circle of support and involve all the people who the person identifies as important to them.

Person-centred planning is about empowering an individual to take control of their life and is a document that is their own and not the professionals.

Implementation of person-centred plan

Five key features are recognised for good person-centred planning and should be used when guiding an individual through a process.

1 *The person is at the centre*: People with learning disabilitie's lives are often controlled by others and they are directed about what they do, what they eat and even what they say. However, person-centred planning aims to address this and provide the individual more dignity and control over their lives. If someone is at the centre of their care, they are the most important person and should be empowered to make decisions in their lives.

2 *Family members and friends are partners in planning*: Family members and friends are often the people that know an individual best and person-centred planning is based on the assumption that the families and friends know what is in the best interest of an individual, even if this best interest is a different view to others. Person-centred planning is about supporting someone to be part of their community and accessing the people who are important in their lives. Families' and friends' views can often help people to develop their plans and can provide their side of an individual's story with a depth that can help individual identify changes.

3 *The plan shows what is important to the person and reflects their capabilities and what support they need*: Person-centred planning is not about focusing on an individual's impairment but on their strengths and capabilities. A person-centred plan should create a consideration of what is important to the person, their aspirations and choices and what support they will need. The person should take the lead.

4 *The plan helps the person be part of their community and shows what is possible – resulting in action*: The focus of person-centred planning is to create an individualised approach and is about everyone working together to make things happen. This includes opening up the local community and helping them be more involved, as communities are diverse and will also benefit from that individual's capacities and strengths. Most important is what sort of life the person wants and enabling this to be in reach.

5 *Everyone keeps on listening, learning and making things happen*: The person-centred plan helps the person achieve what they want from life. Person-centred planning is something that changes with experiences and this means the support may need changing in order to help the person look forward to their future.

Tools

There are several approaches, styles and tools that can be used for person-centred planning, but the one consistent principle is that the plans are based on focusing on the person. Here are some common examples:
- Essential lifestyle planning
- PATHS
- MAPS
- Personal futures planning
- One page profiles.

Although there are many more styles to add to this list, it is important to recognise that these tools are to be adapted to meet the person's needs. The tools are also evolving documents and a good plan would use what is necessary to keep it current. The person centred plans can be created in meetings or as one-to-one support work. One important note is that person-centred planning can take time and individuals may need to focus on some aspects of their lives more than others at different times.

Role of the learning disability nurse

Learning disability nurses have a number of skills that mean they are suited to working in a person-centred way, such as listening, observing and thinking creatively.

Person centred plans are a way for an individual to gain confidence in their own skills and capabilities. Learning disability nurses should aim to guide an individual to set goals and plans and help them to achieve these.

Learning disability nurses who are supporting an individual must always make themselves aware of the individual's person-centred plan. The learning disability nurse's care plan needs to be mindful of the goals set out in the individual's person-centred plan, and be striving to support the individual to achieve these goals. The learning disability nurse is not usually the person best placed to help someone write their person centred plan, as this is usually the individual with their carer, family members or other people in their support network. The learning disability nurse can provide invaluable contributions though, especially with regards to an individual's health and wellbeing.

At times, it can be difficult to help facilitate person centred plans when involving individuals with higher support needs. For individuals with higher support needs, it is extra important to use the five features above to really support the individual and be creative to make the person-centred plan worthwhile.

As the Figure above shows, person-centred planning can be effective and worthwhile for an individual.

Summary

- Person-centred planning can change individual's lives and should be at the heart of all the support learning disability nurses and learning disabilities services can provide.
- Person centred planning is also a way to implement change for individuals and develop ways to be creative and effective when working alongside individuals.
- Most importantly, person centred planning is the chance to really open the community and opportunities for individuals and make their lives as rewarding and fulfilling as they want them to be.

58 Employment

(a) Types of employment support

Work preparation schemes	This could be provided in a college, day service or work placement and involves developing pre-requisite skills required for employment such as time keeping, personal appearance at work and problem solving.
Work experience	Work experience can be provided via a supported employment scheme, voluntary work or in the open marketplace. These are normally supported by schemes such as Shaw Trust or other government commission organisations. These are not normally paid positions and should be time limited to allow the person to develop their skills, experience and confidence for paid employment.
Job coaching	A job coach is a non-disabled person who is assigned to work with the person with a learning disability to help them learn the job. This could be an external person or someone already employed in the organisation.
Working with employers to comply with the Disability Discrimination Act 1995	There are schemes which work with employers to help them understand the individual needs of people with learning disabilities and make appropriate reasonable adjustments.

(b) Common types of employment

Paid
A job with a contract and financial reward. This has the highest value in society.

Unpaid
A job which plays an important supporting role in maintaining society despite the worker not being paid.

Substitute
Work that is contrived for disabled people in a segregated environment such as a sheltered workshop. This is at odds with the social inclusion agenda.

(c) Historical perspective

Outline of historical developments associated with the concept of employment of people with learning disabilities over the years

Institutions
In the first part of the twentieth century, the predominant understanding of learning disability led us to believe that people could not develop skills or meaningfully contribute to society.

Industrial therapy
In the 1960s and 70s the concept of 'normalisation' challenged this view, and the idea of habilitation was introduced into many institutions. Industrial therapy became popular. This was very low-paid, repetitive work such as packing and sorting. It occurred in the hospital setting, but did provide a small wage and a sense of achievement and mastery, which is important to self-esteem.

Sheltered workshops
As policy developed, there was a move to greater community living. In the 1980s people started to move out of the hospital setting. Sheltered work schemes were developed in the community setting. Again, this was usually low-paid and repetitive work. Although based in the community they were still segregated units, only for people with learning disabilities.

Real jobs for real people
In the late 1990s and into the twenty-first century there has been a greater aspiration towards people being supported into real jobs on the open market. There are a range of schemes to support this. Although there remain difficulties in achieving this goal, the drive is towards people doing jobs which they choose and enjoy, and support of integration within wider society.

Learning Disability Nursing at a Glance, First Edition. Edited by Bob Gates, Debra Fearns and Jo Welch. © 2015 John Wiley & Sons, Ltd. Published 2015 by John Wiley & Sons, Ltd.
Companion website: www.ataglanceseries.com/nursing/learningdisability

Introduction

Not everyone wants to be employed, but almost all want to "work", that is to be engaged in some kind of valued activity that uses their skills and facilitates social inclusion. (College of Occupational Therapists and Department of Health, 2007)

Work makes up an important part of our wellbeing. It is widely acknowledged that employment not only has financial benefits but psychosocial benefits too. It helps us develop self-esteem, provides a structure to our time, offers opportunities for social contact and in many cases allows us to develop our skills and obtain a sense of achievement. Many believe that leisure and work are inextricably linked, that is, to truly appreciate leisure and relaxation time we must also have experienced productivity. Unfortunately this has been an area that has been lacking for many people with learning disabilities. The Healthcare Commission 2009 found that despite efforts to get people into employment, very few achieved this. Figure (b) above shows the different types of employment available to people with learning disabilities, very few achieve paid work, some achieve unpaid or substitute work but many do not achieve even these areas of work.

The current situation

'In England, only 6.4 per cent of people with moderate to severe learning disabilities known to adult social services are in paid employment (NHS Information Centre, Social Care and Mental Health Indicators from the National Indicator Set, England 2009-10, August 2010). This is far lower than the employment rate for all disabled people (47.4 per cent) and the working age population in England (77.3 per cent) (Labor Force Survey, quarter 2, 2009).'

Valuing Employment was published in 2009 with the intention of tackling this inequality. It states that employment should no longer be seen as an optional extra for people with learning disabilities. We should develop an expectation of employment and people should be afforded choice about what kind of work they want to do. This paper advocates paid employment on the open market.

Barriers to employment

There are number of reasons why people with learning disabilities find it hard to obtain paid employment. These include:

- Stigmatising views of employers, the general public and in some cases those that support them.
- Difficulty with the necessary literacy skills required to find employment and apply for a job.
- Poor understanding of the needs of people with learning disabilities.
- Difficulty with problem solving and prioritising.
- Fear of failure and poor confidence.
- Slower to learn new skills.
- Difficulty understanding the unspoken social rules.

Making reasonable adjustments to the work environment

The Disability Discrimination Act 1995, and more recently the Equalities Act 2010, make it illegal to discriminate against any person with a disability looking for or in employment. For many people this means making changes to the physical environment, such as ramps and special chairs, and for some it means more flexible working hours; but for someone with a learning disability adjustments may need to be more complex and will be very individual. Reasonable adjustments may mean a greater use of accessible information, taking the time to demonstrate new things and explicitly explain what is expect both for the job and socially within the environment.

How can we help people with learning disabilities gain employment?

There are currently a range of schemes aimed at improving employment opportunities for people with learning disabilities. Figure (a) above describes a few.

The job centre employs Disability Employment Advisors (DEA) who act as gate keepers for these schemes. People can refer themselves; call your local Jobcentre Plus for contact details of your DEA.

What are the advantages of employing someone with a learning disability?

Whilst there are a range of obstacles which make employment more difficult for someone with a learning disability to achieve, it is important to acknowledge that they may bring strengths that others would not. Although these will be very individual they may include:

- A willingness and desire to do repetitive jobs which others find boring.
- Ability to pay attention to detail.
- Less likely to get involved in social politics.
- Desire for routines and therefore greater likelihood to stick to break times and start/finish times.

59 Housing and leisure

Residential alternatives

Hospital accommodation
Retains nursing and medical staff and therapists, and provides a specialist focus of care

Hostels
Often referred to as 'half-way houses' and usually run by social service departments

Supported living
Taking services to the person's own home, and developing around them the kinds of support needed for living as independently as possible

Types of residential alternatives for people with learning disabilities

Family placement
Care within a family other than the person's own, as an alternative to residential care

Intentional communities
An inclusive term for cohousing communities, residential land trusts, communes, student co-ops, urban housing co-operatives, co-operative living, and other projects where people strive together with a common vision

Village communities
Residents contribute what they can to the wellbeing of other members according to their ability

Leisure alternatives

Leisure is important to everyone's mental health and sense of wellbeing, and this is also true for people with learning disabilities

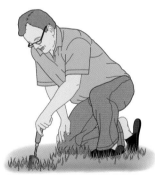

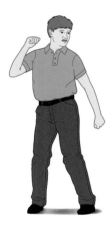

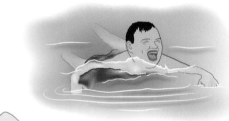

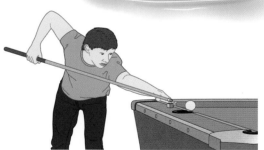

In providing leisure facilities, the learning disability nurse needs to consider:

- Transport
- Costs
- Accessible facilities
- It is important to make sure that careful plans are in place

Learning Disability Nursing at a Glance, First Edition. Edited by Bob Gates, Debra Fearns and Jo Welch. © 2015 John Wiley & Sons, Ltd. Published 2015 by John Wiley & Sons, Ltd.
Companion website: www.ataglanceseries.com/nursing/learningdisability

Introduction

In most Western countries, residential care and leisure activities for people with learning disabilities have been influenced by political, ideological and economic factors, and have developed in parallel paths. But given that people with learning disabilities have been, and still are, often misunderstood, these paths have sometimes resulted in inappropriate residential care and leisure opportunities being offered to them and their families. Today, the preferred living arrangement for most people is supported living, and the preferred leisure activities reside in the use of inclusive community based resources.

Residential alternatives
Hospital type accommodation

Despite the closure of most of the long-stay learning disability hospitals, some residential care provision, known as 'residential campuses', has remained. Generally speaking, this type of provision retains nursing and medical staff and therapists, and provides a specialist focus of care.

Hostels

Hostels emerged during the 1960s and 1970s. Typically they catered for approximately 12–30 people, were often referred to as 'half-way houses' and were usually run by social service departments. Many of these establishments remained institutionalised, and continued to perpetuate systems of block treatment and depersonalised forms of care. A development of the provision of hostel accommodation was that of 'core and cluster' arrangements where a number of smaller, 'ordinary' houses were clustered around a larger residential unit.

Family placements for adults

Adult placements evolved from the fostering of children with special needs from the 1970s. There are many adult family placement schemes to be found across the countries of the UK and the Republic of Ireland. People with learning disabilities are placed in families other than their own, as an alternative to residential care; the families are approved and trained by an official agency.

Village communities

The origins of these communities lie in the Camphill Village movement, established by Dr Karl König. This movement is based on the educational theories of Rudolf Steiner (1861–1925), and it was from his philosophy that the idea of therapeutic communities developed. Such communities are designed to; 'foster the harmonious development of the whole human being – body, soul and spirit – to create a healthy balance between thinking, feeling, and with activity and to engender morality, social co-operation and responsibility'. In these communities, residents contribute what they can to the wellbeing of other members according to their abilities.

Intentional communities

Village communities sometimes get muddled with intentional communities; the term community means more than a small village configuration of residencies. Other types of residential community include L'Arche, a federation of communities in the UK, France, Denmark, Belgium, Norway and the USA as well as in India and the Cottage and Rural Enterprise and the Home Farm Trust.

Supported living and home ownership

Supported living might best be thought of not as a single model, but as a range of residential alternatives for people with learning disabilities; however, central to all alternatives are living in one's own home and participating in one's own community. Supported living was developed in the USA and was born from frustration with the dominant residential alternatives for people with learning disabilities. Supported living represents a way of constructing services that takes services to people's own homes, and then develops around them the kinds of support that they need to live as independently as possible.

Leisure alternatives

In the past, leisure for people with learning disabilities was provided in segregated places such as day centres. Today people with learning disabilities try and access the same kind and range of leisure activities that all citizens enjoy. Leisure refers to the time we spend doing things that we enjoy. It includes a wide variety of activities, for example sports, art, reading, sewing, stamp and coin collecting. Leisure is important to our mental health and wellbeing, and this is also true of people with learning disabilities. However, finding accessible leisure activities for people with learning disabilities can be a challenge. For this group of people there are some important things to remember and these include; transport, costs and accessible facilities. For learning disability nurses it is important to make sure that careful plans are made to ensure people with learning disabilities get involved in leisure activities on their own, and with their friends and or family. Recently Emerson and Hatton (2008) identified the kinds of leisure activities that people with learning disabilities were engaged in. They reported, 'that those with profound and multiple learning disabilities were. . . less likely to participate in a range of leisure and community-based activities than people with mild/moderate or severe learning disabilities'. Activities included: shopping, visiting friends or family, eating out in a restaurant, pub or café, going to the pub or club, going to the hairdresser, playing sport or going swimming, going to the cinema, going to a play or concert, visiting the library, watching sport.

Summary
- Despite the closure of most long-stay hospitals for people with learning disabilities, some 'residential campuses' have remained, providing specialist care.
- There are a range of housing provisions for people with learning disabilities, ranging from living with family/parents to supported living.
- Leisure facilities have improved accessibility for people with learning disabilities, but challenges may still remain due to transport and travel costs.

60 Ethnic minorities and learning disability

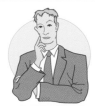

When working with people with a learning disability from ethnic minority backgrounds:

- Be aware of barriers to health, social care and education
- Challenge institutional racism
- Be sensitive to people's culture
- Do not generalise and make assumptions about people. Ask how you can support them

What is ethnicity?

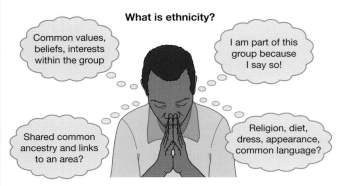

Common values, beliefs, interests within the group

I am part of this group because I say so!

Shared common ancestry and links to an area?

Religion, diet, dress, appearance, common language?

Cultural Sensitivity

Be aware that different groups of people have different views and beliefs. Be sensitive to the following:

Modesty and privacy	Food preferences
Clothing, jewellery, make-up	Family
Washing, hygiene	Physical examination
Hair and skin care	Birth and birth control (contraception)
Prayer	Death
Holy days and festivals	Medication
Ritual	Organ donation/transplant

Learning Disability Nursing at a Glance, First Edition. Edited by Bob Gates, Debra Fearns and Jo Welch. © 2015 John Wiley & Sons, Ltd. Published 2015 by John Wiley & Sons, Ltd.
Companion website: www.ataglanceseries.com/nursing/learningdisability

Introduction

The United Kingdom is regarded as one of the most ethnically diverse countries in the world. According to the 2001 census, 8% of the population (4.6 million) were from a minority ethnic group.

Higher prevalence of learning difficulties can be found in several ethnic groups. This has been linked to high levels of material and social deprivation. These combine with other factors, such as poor access to maternal healthcare, misclassification and higher rates of environmental or genetic risk factors.

As a nurse you will need to work with people from ethnic minorities or cultures different from your own. These people may be service users, families or fellow staff members. People from ethnic minority backgrounds need support that is culturally sensitive and appropriate for their needs.

What is ethnicity?

Ethnicity is the preferred term to describe race and culture. It is a fluid term used by individuals to assert their identity at any point in life.

Barriers to health, social care and education and inequality

Many families and people with learning disabilities who are from minority ethnic groups are unaware of the extent of learning disability services. Problems are made worse when professionals are unaware of the cultural, religious and language needs of ethnic groups.

For example, letters may be sent to carers in a language that the carer or person with a learning disability cannot understand. Medical appointments may be made during religious holidays; culturally appropriate food may not be available to people using services. Often carers do not know where to access services. A lack of knowledge about other people and services can produce mistrust amongst people from perspectives of both the person from a minority group and the service givers. Minority ethnic communities and people with learning disabilities both face substantial inequalities and discrimination in employment, education, health and social services. There is a link between poor health and poorer socio-economic conditions.

Institutional racism

It is important that we challenge institutional racism if we come across it:

Institutional racism consists of the collective failure of an organisation to provide an appropriate and professional service to people because of their colour, culture or ethnic origin. It can be seen or detected in processes, attitudes and behaviour which amount to discrimination through unwitting prejudice, ignorance, thoughtlessness and racial stereotyping, which disadvantage ethnic minority people.
(The Stephen Lawrence Inquiry, 1999)

Ways to support people with a learning disability from a ethnic minority

- Use plain English language, not complex medical jargon.
- Use the service user's first language if possible.
- Written or pictorial information around health interventions explaining the processes.
- Communicating about your services and health issues with places of worship and community centres.
- Use of translation services rather than family members.
- Be aware of appointment times. Some religious groups may need to pray or will not be able to use transport after sundown on religious days. It is vital you understand this and allow for appointment times that are sensitive to people's beliefs.
- Same sex professionals to work with clients. Some families and service users may request a carer or nurse of the same sex not just for intimate care but other forms of support.
- Hair, skin and clothing care might be different from your own.
- A person may wish for someone of their own ethnicity to work with them. Respect their choice. Alternatively they may wish for someone outside their community in order to respect their privacy and increase confidentiality. Be aware that you will be sharing information of a sensitive nature.
- Food choices need to be culturally sensitive: it is a matter of individual interpretation of a person's own culture as to how they define their ethnicity. Always ask the person.
- Try to think outside your own culture by reflecting on your own values and where they come from. Just because you do something one way does not mean others have to or that it is right.
- All your service users should have a hospital passport and person-centred plan. These should detail any religious and ethnic needs to the person's care.
- Establish contacts within the communities you work with and build positive links with them.
- Empower and support families, carers and individuals with personal budgets and direct payments. This will enable them to tailor care to the cultural needs of the service user and family.

Always personalise support and care. Ask the service user how you can support them using person centred approaches.

61 Parents with a learning disability

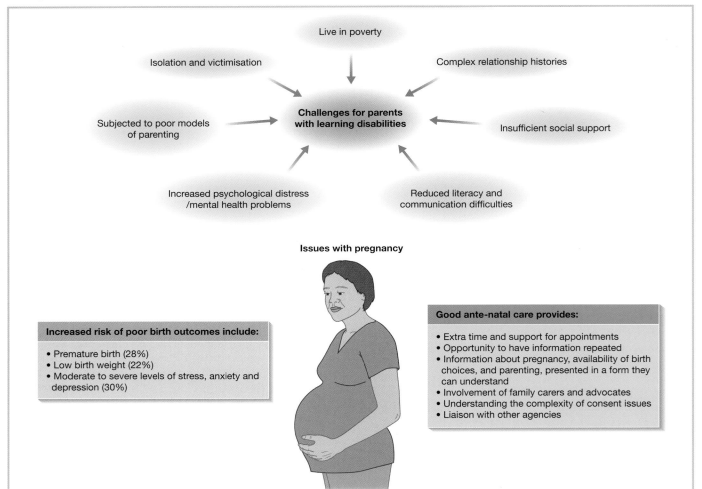

Live in poverty

Isolation and victimisation

Complex relationship histories

Challenges for parents with learning disabilities

Subjected to poor models of parenting

Insufficient social support

Increased psychological distress /mental health problems

Reduced literacy and communication difficulties

Issues with pregnancy

Increased risk of poor birth outcomes include:

- Premature birth (28%)
- Low birth weight (22%)
- Moderate to severe levels of stress, anxiety and depression (30%)

Good ante-natal care provides:

- Extra time and support for appointments
- Opportunity to have information repeated
- Information about pregnancy, availability of birth choices, and parenting, presented in a form they can understand
- Involvement of family carers and advocates
- Understanding the complexity of consent issues
- Liaison with other agencies

Learning Disability Nursing at a Glance, First Edition. Edited by Bob Gates, Debra Fearns and Jo Welch. © 2015 John Wiley & Sons, Ltd. Published 2015 by John Wiley & Sons, Ltd.
Companion website: www.ataglanceseries.com/nursing/learningdisability

*P*eople with learning disabilities can be good parents and provide their children with a good start in life, but may require considerable help to do so. (Government Consultation, 2007)

Many concerns have been discussed triggering debate and anxiety regarding people with a learning disability becoming parents. Frequently, pregnant women with learning disabilities have faced criticism and judgement, often being subjected to the beliefs and attitudes of those around them. This is based in much controversy between the reality and perception of those supporting the parents.

People with learning disabilities face opposition to their desire to parent or alarm at the announcement of a pregnancy- some parents face pressure for a termination.

Typically, parents with learning disabilities:
- are living in poverty
- are isolated and victimised
- have been subjected to poor models of parenting
- have difficult relationship histories
- receive insufficient social support
- have increased psychological distress/mental health problems
- have reduced literacy
- experience communication difficulties.

All of these will impact upon their ability to cope with the demands of raising children. However it is evident that services do not necessarily look beyond the label of 'learning disability' and tend to neglect the complexity of factors that influence parental competence.

Since Valuing People (DoH, 2001), the focus of the work alongside people with a learning disability has been towards leading ordinary lives, and this includes being a parent. There is much prejudice against people with learning disabilities and this is especially the situation when they or think about becoming parents, with as many as 30–40% of parents with learning disabilities having children removed. There is little support set up to discuss this, although Valuing People Now (DoH, 2009) gives some clarity regarding the way things need to change. This necessitates fundamental change in services reviewing the way they work, so that parents and their children receive the support they are entitled to. The right support at the right time could mean that fewer parents with learning disabilities have their children removed. The right support could enable parents and their children to stay together safely as a family as a right under the Human Rights Act (1998). Around 7% of adults with a learning disability have become parents, but most have a mild to borderline leaning disability, which may make it difficult to identify them as they may not have a formal diagnosis and are often not in receipt of services. The children of parents with a learning disability are more likely than any other group of children to be removed from their parents' care. This should not be the case.

- Valuing People Now (DoH, 2009) states that people with learning disability should have the choice to have relationships, become parents, continue to be parents and be supported to do so.
- Services need to support parents with learning disabilities. At the moment parents do not get the support they need and are therefore at risk of enforced separation.
- Adult and children's services need to work together effectively so that there is an integrated system to support people.
- People should receive equitable support from all mainstream family services, should have access to advocacy and the same level of information and advice as everyone else considering reasonable adjustments.

All partnership boards should make sure parents with learning disabilities have accessible information services and individual budgets to support families. The Government has also written Good Practice Guidance on working with parents with learning disabilities (DoH, 2007) for professionals.

Issues in pregnancy

The babies of mothers with learning disabilities are at increased risk of poor birth outcomes, including:
- Premature birth (28%)
- Low birth weight (22%)
- Moderate to severe levels of stress, anxiety and depression (30%).

Issues for ante-natal care and education

Women with a learning disability are more likely to have difficulty in accessing good quality ante-natal care that meets their needs, including:
- extra time and support for appointments
- opportunity to have information repeated
- information about pregnancy, availability of birth choices and parenting that is presented in an empowering form that they can understand
- involvement of family carers and advocates
- understanding the complexity of consent issues
- liaison with other agencies involved.

Some women with a learning disability may avoid maternity care because of lack of confidence, negative staff attitudes, lack of clear explanations of what is going on, inaccessible leaflets, and fear of the involvement of social services. Ante-natal education is vital for parents with a learning disability who may find themselves having their parental competence assessed soon after birth by social workers, before they have had time to develop and practise their skills and confidence as parents. However, most parents with learning disabilities do not access mainstream ante-natal classes, and might benefit from tailored classes or individual ante-natal education.

To be inclusive, ante-natal classes could:
- work to be enabling and empowering
- focus on building the opportunity to gain confidence, develop skills and make meaningful relationships
- be facilitated with a positive focus/attitude
- present information in accessible formats which relate to the parents
- provide visual resources and use plain English
- provide opportunities to try out practical skills more than once
- use role play and modelling
- talk to other parents with a positive experience
- empower the transfer of skills learnt to new and different situations.

It is vital to get to know the parents and children from the beginning of the relationship, in order to build trust, confidence and belief in each other and to agree on ways of working together and how to maintain contact. This may be different for each family. It is important to build information about the ways and means people learn, for example is it easier to learn something new by being shown or by doing it with someone.

Gaining a greater insight into the family and the children ensures a greater understanding of their situation and how their family operates. Working in this way may facilitate the development of new strategies, for example time and changing domestic routines, and gaining a greater awareness of the priorities of the family, what can be achieved, what cannot and how they interact with the children.

It is imperative that there is a move away from the negative assumptions, attitudes and barriers frequently experienced by parents with a learning disability, as they face the struggles of being a parent and being 'good enough' for their children in the eyes of those around them. A proactive approach to supporting parents and ensuring a positive outcome for the family is the way forward, thus ensuring equitable treatment for parents with learning disabilities.

62 Family perspectives

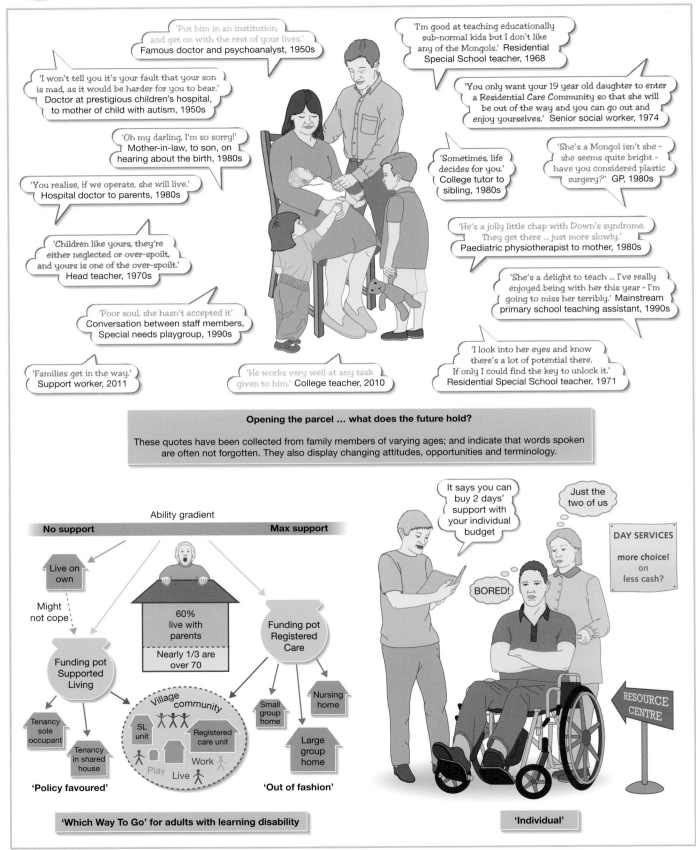

'Put him in an institution, and get on with the rest of your lives.'
Famous doctor and psychoanalyst, 1950s

'I'm good at teaching educationally sub-normal kids but I don't like any of the Mongols.' Residential Special School teacher, 1968

'I won't tell you it's your fault that your son is mad, as it would be harder for you to bear.' Doctor at prestigious children's hospital, to mother of child with autism, 1950s

'You only want your 19 year old daughter to enter a Residential Care Community so that she will be out of the way and you can go out and enjoy yourselves.' Senior social worker, 1974

'Oh my darling, I'm so sorry!' Mother-in-law, to son, on hearing about the birth, 1980s

'Sometimes, life decides for you.' College tutor to sibling, 1980s

'She's a Mongol isn't she - she seems quite bright - have you considered plastic surgery?' GP, 1980s

'You realise, if we operate, she will live.' Hospital doctor to parents, 1980s

'He's a jolly little chap with Down's syndrome. They get there ... just more slowly.' Paediatric physiotherapist to mother, 1980s

'Children like yours, they're either neglected or over-spoilt, and yours is one of the over-spoilt.' Head teacher, 1970s

'She's a delight to teach ... I've really enjoyed being with her this year - I'm going to miss her terribly.' Mainstream primary school teaching assistant, 1990s

'Poor soul, she hasn't accepted it' Conversation between staff members, Special needs playgroup, 1990s

'I look into her eyes and know there's a lot of potential there. If only I could find the key to unlock it.' Residential Special School teacher, 1971

'Families get in the way.' Support worker, 2011

'He works very well at any task given to him.' College teacher, 2010

Opening the parcel … what does the future hold?

These quotes have been collected from family members of varying ages; and indicate that words spoken are often not forgotten. They also display changing attitudes, opportunities and terminology.

Ability gradient

No support — **Max support**

Live on own

Might not cope

Funding pot Supported Living

60% live with parents

Nearly 1/3 are over 70

Funding pot Registered Care

Nursing home

Small group home

Large group home

Tenancy sole occupant

Tenancy in shared house

Village community

SL unit

Registered care unit

Play · Work · Live

'Policy favoured'

'Out of fashion'

It says you can buy 2 days' support with your individual budget

Just the two of us

DAY SERVICES more choice! on less cash?

BORED!

RESOURCE CENTRE

'Which Way To Go' for adults with learning disability

'Individual'

Learning Disability Nursing at a Glance, First Edition. Edited by Bob Gates, Debra Fearns and Jo Welch. © 2015 John Wiley & Sons, Ltd. Published 2015 by John Wiley & Sons, Ltd.
Companion website: www.ataglanceseries.com/nursing/learningdisability

Some family perspectives

All of us start life within a family of some sort, even if, very rarely, we lose contact later. The family is considered a basic building block of society and culture, but takes many different forms. However if your family also includes someone who is described as having 'learning disabilities' this presents unique challenges, and often lifelong stresses and concerns.

Rising to these challenges can bring great satisfaction, and professionals such as learning disability nurses can provide vital help. Recognising that the family is usually the most important, consistent and reliably helpful resource in a learning disabled person's life is essential, as is the understanding that these families often face a lifelong struggle to support their loved one. Those without families willing to do this on their behalf are doubly disadvantaged.

Words we use

Good communication underlies good understanding, but words often get in the way. The current labels 'learning disabilities' and 'learning difficulties' and 'special needs' are regarded by many families to be almost meaningless, covering a wide range of circumstances; a person can be almost completely independent, or need constant support to do even the most basic tasks, including self-care, and there is everything in between.

Families experience learning disabilities often within a complex of other needs, as the conditions which give rise to them vary widely, affecting many aspects of a person's ability to function. Everyone is unique. Many families also feel that rejecting the 'disability' label altogether in favour of 'difficulties' downplays the real impact of the condition.

Starting out

Babies are usually welcomed joyfully, but those born with disabilities often present parents and wider family with very conflicted emotions.

Every baby is a parcel you learn to unwrap. (advice given at (non-disabled) pre-natal group)

The care a family provides for a newborn usually lessens as they grow, but if the child has significant disabilities it may need to be lifelong. Families are all unique, and make their own version of 'normal' but the 'normal' for a learning disabled family is often very different. Siblings may become child-carers, a role which follows them into adulthood, have to cope with challenging behaviours, and the family itself may suffer from social exclusion. Considering the needs of siblings and parents and involving both in planning for the person at the centre is essential.

Growing up and moving on

Young adults with learning disabilities can now carry on in full time education until their 20s, if families can get funding from Local Authorities. Afterwards, two thirds of adults with learning disabilities continue to live with their families, often a significant stress on ageing parents, who still continue as long as they can. A lack of services, acceptable accommodation options and funding mean that for many moving on only occurs in a crisis. Parents often find they fall over a cliff edge in service provision after they leave education funding.

Families, services and official government policy

Families still often feel 'at the receiving end', lacking time or energy to lobby. However, historically, families have been very involved in campaigning; creating and running many well-known voluntary organisations which provide services, such as MENCAP.

Most current policy arose first in the context of physical disability and a rejection of attitudes which primarily view disabled people as patients; 'the medical model of disability'. Many families recognise that although society often makes the experience of disability much worse, 'the social model of disability' in the case of learning disabilities, medical expertise is still needed and often sadly lacking.

The idea that we see the person first, not the disability, has led to approaches such as 'person-centred planning' which should always involve families as partners. A reaction against earlier institutionalisation now promotes services based in 'the community' and an assertion of 'choice'. However, the practical consequence has been a move away from traditional services. 'Normalisation', originally an idea that having a disability is just part of the normal range of 'being human', has been interpreted as 'mainstreaming'. that is that persons with disabilities can just use facilities used by the mainstream population, 'out in the community'. (*Why do you need a Day Centre, if you can go to a coffee shop?*) Many families recognise that dedicated services are still needed, and function better if they have a permanent building.

Another new idea, personal budgets, should allow people to choose how their support money is spent. However, if they lack capacity to do this themselves, there are restrictions on how it can be spent, or it is inadequate in amount, a policy which improves things for some may place increased burdens on others, especially if the changes mean losing day centre or respite places. Additionally, using standard assessment procedures, which focus on age related or physical disabilities, it is often difficult to communicate the particular aspects which families consider make learning disabilities far more 'disabling' than commonly recognised. It is often an 'invisible' disability, which only reveals itself fully when 'tested' in a social situation.

Summary
- Families usually have the best, lifelong understanding of the person, and are the most constant presence in their lives.
- Challenging behaviours are usually caused by a failure of communication or failure to meet needs, not mental health issues.
- Always take guidance from the Mental Capacity Act first, not the Mental Health Act.
- Health needs of persons with learning disabilities, including mental health needs, are often unmet, even when the person is perceived as very 'able'. This is because individuals often do not speak up for themselves, families may be overwhelmed, and problems may be wrongly attributed to the underlying 'learning disability' rather than investigated properly for a medical cause.
- Siblings of any age are often helpful but often left out.

63 A service user's perspective

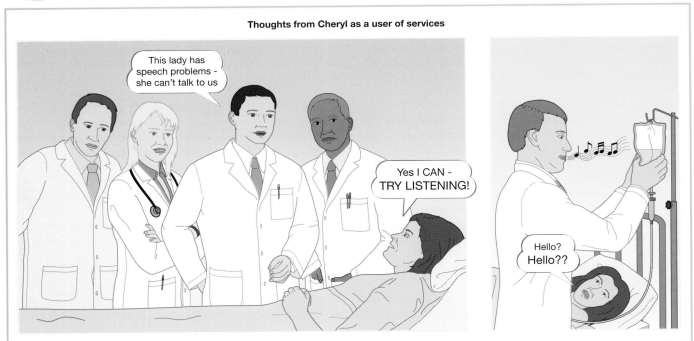

Treat people with learning difficulties/disabilities like anybody else where possible.

'Some time ago I went to my Doctors, and I told him that I was in severe pain and, basically, he told me I was "a Hypochondriac – the pain was all in my head". At the time I looked 9 months pregnant – at that time it was not realised how sick I actually was. My whole system was shutting down. The doctor was treating me like an imbecile, but another GP took action immediately and referred me to the hospital. I do not know if that was because I had a friend with me or not – at the time I didn't care.'

When I went in hospital, how I was treated.

'I was appalled at how little they knew about physical disability and learning disability, and how to care for my needs. I was asked to go into the day room because "I was in the way". Out of sight – out of mind! I felt isolated, like my wellbeing was not exactly a priority. I was an object with a mental age of 5. I felt pissed off. Felt like a bag of potatoes, talked to like a child. One doctor wanted to put me through more unnecessary pain by fitting me with a stoma bag! My response was "I am not old before my time – NO thank you" (in a polite way). The staff were talking amongst themselves, over my bed, as if I was not present, and what really pissed me off; they waited for friends and family members to do personal care, even when it was a male friend. So I felt even more undervalued as a person, no self-worth. THEN the registrar came in my room and started to treat me like a Human Being, not like an object, and he explained, in a clear and simple way so I could understand what was happening to me, and he also told me that "If we don't start the bowel moving NOW then the whole system will be poisoned". At that point I was shitting myself (figuratively – the whole problem was that I wasn't!) because I knew what he was saying about my prognosis. He went against his colleague and tried an alternative approach – which worked!'

Knowing people.

'Where the learning disability (LD) is too severe to allow the patient to meaningfully speak for themselves then use an advocate, if necessary involve other services that work with LD. I would like a person who knew me personally and that I could trust, this does not necessarily mean a family member. I have a friend who has got a rare multiplicity of conditions, and if you don't know her well enough, and understand her pain and intense frustration, she can get emotional and have physical outbursts, screaming and biting her hand, pulling her hair. I have been told that the mother and carers need to do her care in hospital, because she cannot communicate her needs to those who don't know her. She has recently had rods put in her back. The mother had to drive 30 miles each way each day to provide care and reassurance with lots of cuddles. From her point of view it was confusing, frightening and very distressing and isolating. This happened to coincide with her moving house as well, adding to the distress.'

How do we know we are using the right service for an individual, when they can't voice their opinions?

'I have known several people, with moderate LD, living independently, but with very painful conditions (e.g. Crohn's, pancreatitis) that got so frustrated at not being listened to or explained to that they turned to alcohol to try and numb the pain. This got them telling offs and they became frightened of even going to hospital, I know one of them missed appointment after appointment and has got into a painful downward spiral of pain and drink. I was involved in a recent situation where a severe LD patient was very sick but no one, doctors, nurses, parents could get the patient to tell them what was wrong. Only after we had got everyone out of the room, and I could clam her down and talk to her gently, with sign language, would she explain the problem.'

What do services need to do – a check list – at least as I see it as a service user.

- 'LISTEN! Listen to the patient – however difficult the speech may be. Don't ignore parents/carers BUT listen.
- Do a risk assessment.
- As far as possible, all written information should be in easy read or similar formats so the patient can understand them.
- Try to be near to the patient's level, if possible sit by the bed and try and maintain eye contact.
- All involved nurses and staff should have appropriate disability awareness training and be empathetic towards LD patients.
- Be careful about labelling! Labels can be very useful, but inappropriate ones can cause much harm.'

What about learning disability liaison nurses?

'A good, properly trained, LD liaison nurse, who is empathetic to his/her patient, and who has the patience to learn how to understand that patient, and is given time to build trust and mutual respect with that patient, may be able to reduce the need for external involvement, so enabling appropriate treatment to take place more effectively and quickly. To do their job most effectively they must also have the respect and trust of the other ward staff. They should also play a valuable role in advising other ward staff on how to work with and treat the LD patient.'

Care planning – who controls it?

'Care planning' is essential, but if the care recipient cannot, for whatever reason, tell you what they want, and only trusts close friends, and possibly an advocate, neither of whom may be involved in the process, it may not meet their needs. A close friend of mine had all his care planning done for him by his mother. The friend was only mildly LD, more difficulty than disability, but the family chose to treat him as being moderate to severe LD, incapable of making his own decisions, or even deciding what he liked or didn't. Even when he moved to an independent house this continued. As his confidence built he was able to start being involved in, and then controlling, his own care planning. If he needs help he asks for it.'

64 Advocacy

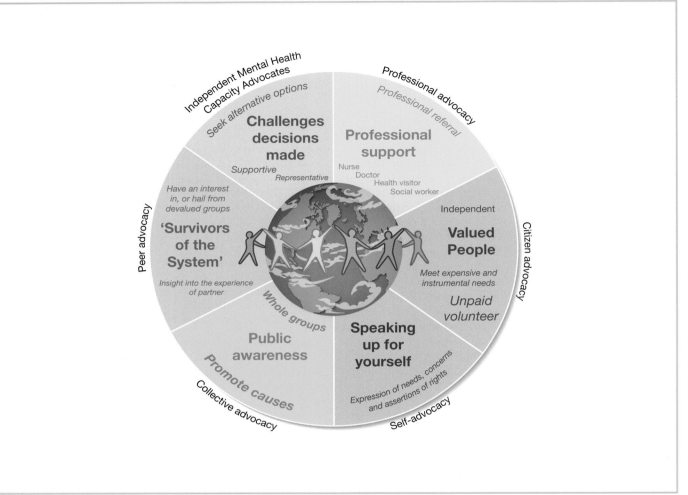

Introduction

Advocacy is fundamentally concerned with speaking up for oneself as in self-advocacy, or with others in a group, or through collective advocacy, as well as through others in citizen or peer advocacy (Atkinson, 1999). Therefore, a basic definition of advocacy is '*speaking for oneself or on behalf of others*'.

Advocacy is associated with a number of types of representation including: self; an unpaid person (such as a friend, relative or citizen advocate); a paid person (perhaps a community nurse or social worker); or organisation such as People First or MENCAP.

Self-advocacy

Self-advocacy is practised by many of us as individuals but groups can provide a good setting for developing self-advocacy skills, particularly for people who are at risk of being devalued in society. Self-advocacy has great potential to enhance the lives of people with learning disabilities as they become more aware of rights, express needs and concerns and assert interests. Self-advocacy has been described as the ultimate goal of all other forms of advocacy (Atkinson, 1999). Definitions of self-advocacy often include 'speaking up for yourself' but making decisions, taking action, and changing things are significant components which self-advocacy groups have identified. According to Crawley (1988), self-advocacy is 'the act of making choices and decisions and bringing about desired change for oneself. Any activity that involves self-determination can be called self-advocacy'. Self-advocacy is inclusive – all can be involved. 'Everyone can take part in self-advocacy at some level regardless of the severity of their disabilities' (Crawley, 1988).

Citizen advocacy

This refers to a supportive partnership from a volunteer with a relationship with a person who is vulnerable to being disadvantaged through illness, age or disability. It is important that advocates are 'valued people', that is not themselves disadvantaged. Advocates form a close personal relationship with their partners, helping them to make choices and decisions. They work independently of services to uphold the rights of their partners as citizens. Citizen advocacy refers to the persuasive and supportive activities of trained, selected volunteers and coordinating staff working on behalf of those who are disabled/disadvantaged and not in a good position to exercise or defend their rights as citizens. Citizen advocates are persons who are independent of those providing direct services to people with disabilities. Working on a one-to-one basis, they attempt to foster respect for the rights and dignity of those they represent. This may involve helping to express the individual's needs and wishes, helping them to access services, and providing practical and emotional support. The benefits of a partnership with a citizen advocate fall into two broad categories according to the nature of the needs met: expressive (human, emotional and social needs) and instrumental (material needs).

Peer advocacy

Individual support provided by someone who is also a member of a section of society that is in danger of being devalued or stigmatised. Thus, a person with a learning disability could be assisted to articulate their needs and wishes by a peer who also has a learning disability. The peer advocate is likely to have more insight into the experience of their partner than a non-disabled advocate would. A key difference between peer and citizen advocacy is that peer advocates are not 'valued persons' but people who are 'survivors of the system' (Brandon, 1995).

Professional advocacy

This has an important role to play in supporting the empowerment of clients. This might involve introduction to a self-advocacy group or to an independent advocacy service.

Collective advocacy

Collective advocacy is about user representation. There is an important nuance here between advocacy and user representation. Self-advocates represent their own interests; citizen advocates uphold the rights of their partners. User oganisations cannot represent each individual's views but they can promote the cause of minority groups, including people with a learning disability, by raising public awareness and lobbying policy makers on their behalf. Key organisations which help to further the cause of people with a learning disability include: MENCAP, People First, BILD (British Institute of Learning Disabilities), and SCOPE.

Independent mental capacity advocates

Recent legislation has important implications for people with a learning disability and in particular these include: the Equality Act 2010, the Mental Capacity Act 2000, and the Human Rights Act 1985. The effect in practice of the Mental Capacity Act 2005 is that capacity must be assumed. The Act provides a two-stage test for capacity. Firstly, it has to be established that a person suffers from an impairment of, or a disturbance in, the functioning of the mind or brain. Furthermore, it must be demonstrated that this impairment or disturbance results in an inability to make decisions (Dimond, 2007).

The Act presumes that each adult has the right to make his own decisions, and that individuals must be given all appropriate help before any conclusion is reached that they do not have the capacity to do this. Other principles of the Act (as well as presumption of capacity) are: the right of the individual to be supported to make their own decisions. People must be provided with all the appropriate help before any conclusion that they cannot make their own decisions. Unwise decisions: an individual is not to be treated as unable to make a decision simply because it is considered unwise. The Mental Health Act (2007) states that the appropriate authority 'must make such arrangements as it considers reasonable' to enable persons ('independent mental capacity advocates') to be available to represent and support persons who fall within the remit of the Act; Sections 35 and 36 deal with the appointment and function of independent mental capacity advocates.

65 Health passports

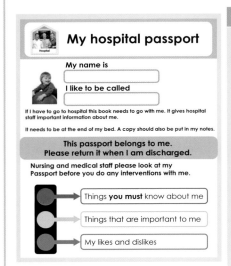

My hospital passport

My name is

I like to be called

If I have to go to hospital this book needs to go with me. It gives hospital staff important information about me.

It needs to be at the end of my bed. A copy should also be put in my notes.

**This passport belongs to me.
Please return it when I am discharged.**

Nursing and medical staff please look at my Passport before you do any interventions with me.

Things **you must** know about me

Things that are important to me

My likes and dislikes

The health passport provides:

- reasonable adjustments for those involved
- flexible response to health needs
- engagement for all people involved
- healthcare staff with a process to make information relevant
- a means to share relevant important information
- personalised adjustments for individuals
- improved health outcomes and experiences
- individuals are more involved in the LD patient's care
- provision of health service in a personalised and dignified manner
- insight into individual's health
- information relevant and timely to individuals
- the ability to act on real-time information
- a means for care and treatment to be delivered equitably
- capacity to be less of a grey area
- a link to communication tools/aids
- reduced inequalities
- a way to meet legal obligations and NHS Outcomes

NHS Outcomes Framework 2014/15 1

Domain 1
Preventing people from dying prematurely

Domain 2
Enhancing quality of life for people with long-term conditions

Domain 3
Helping people to recover from episodes of ill-health or following injury

Domain 4
Ensuring that people have a positive experience of care

Domain 5
Treating and caring for people in a safe environment and protecting them from avoidable harm

What is a health passport

People with a learning disability have greater health needs than the general population. Often they have health needs requiring frequent hospital admission; generally this is twice the average of those who use health services. It is therefore imperative that these needs are given the appropriate support and adjustments and the healthcare workers are enabled to undertake their role in a safe manner. A health passport contains information about the individual which is relevant to their health. This not only provides a picture of the person, it will include information that is about their individual communication, social and behavioural needs. It is important that at all times people complete their own passports and, where help and support is required, this is undertaken with people who know the individual well. This may be family members, carers, advocates, friends or supporters.

The premise is for individuals to own their own passport so they can use it as they need to inform others of health needs and provide information which is timely, systematic in nature and at all times live. The passport should be taken when an individual is due to attend a routine health appointment or an emergency. Even if the passport comes following the emergency, it still has a valuable place.

There are many different health passports which all look and appear different; however, they all will contain similar information. Often individuals will take the opportunity to personalise theirs and add information which they feel is relevant to them.

The main aim of the passport is to ensure that people are increasingly involved in their care and as a result care is more personalised, dignified and safe. This meets the criteria in the NHS Outcomes framework and is an applicable reasonable adjustment.

Passports have made impact and change in the delivery of care for individuals: often the historical information can provide a wider picture of health and overcome often difficult communication barriers, time constraints and repetitive information giving. These will impact on health outcomes and the experience of everyone involved.

This empowering tool enables individuals with a passport and the health professionals involved to make this valuable connection and prevent the differences that exist in the health needs of people with a learning disability. This information will contain solid evidence and information that will prevent healthcare professionals making decisions that are based on assumptions (see Figure above).

Learning Disability Nursing at a Glance, First Edition. Edited by Bob Gates, Debra Fearns and Jo Welch. © 2015 John Wiley & Sons, Ltd. Published 2015 by John Wiley & Sons, Ltd.
Companion website: www.ataglanceseries.com/nursing/learningdisability

...

66 Hate crime

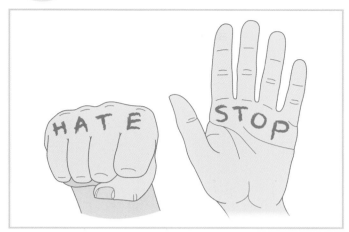

What is hate crime?

Many disabled people feel that their disability is the least of their problems. It is the attitudes and reactions of others to their disability that can cause them most pain. These range from facing prejudice, to being bullied, hassled, ignored and, in some extreme cases, to experiencing hate crime. This chapter examines hate crimes and its impact on individuals, society and how to deal with it as a professional. Let's start by looking at what is a hate crime. It can feature the following: abuse, bullying or antisocial behaviour. It requires two elements to be satisfied: first it must be a criminal act (e.g. theft or arson); and second it must be motivated in whole or in part by the victim's perceived disability status. The police and the Crown Prosecution Service believe that it is a very serious crime. So much so that people who commit disability hate crimes will receive a severe custodial sentence.

Examples of hate crime

This aspect of people's lives, while clearly not new, has for too long been overlooked. The reason it is getting more attention now is that disability groups have very firmly placed it on the agenda. A number of shocking cases have been featured in the media, such as the vicious murder of Brent Martin by three young men. Brent Martin had a learning disability. Martin believed that he was friends with the men, who over the course of time first took his savings, £3000 in total, and then when the money ran out turned on him, killing him in a very cruel manner. In court, the men were found guilty but not under anti-hate crime legislation, the police did go down that route. They got away with a shorter sentence.

Another high-profile case was that of Fiona Pilkington, who was driven to a state of despair by harassment of her and her disabled daughter by teenagers. She reported these incidents to the police a total of 30 times without receiving any response. In despair, she killed herself and her daughter. There have been less high-profile incidents such as targeting and vandalising minibuses for disabilities.

What research tells us

The research literature on the prevalence of hate crime in the learning disability community is very small, it suggests that disabled adults are roughly two to five times more likely to be bullied than non-disabled adults; with people with learning disability being particularly vulnerable. It is difficult to get exact figures at the moment, due to issues around the reporting of crimes by individuals. It seems that the majority are not reported at all. The charity, MENCAP, has been doing work with police forces to improve their response to people with learning disabilities. The police have received training to deal more effectively with these crimes. In some forces they have specialist officers.

The research also tells us that the majority of abuse happens in the home of the person with a disability, and we need to face up to the fact that the main abusers are from their support network. There may be a number of reasons why people with learning disability are vulnerable to hate crimes; it could be they are seen as 'an easy target'. They may feel 'not one of us' or 'an ugly duckling' and as a result develop a poor sense of self. The perpetrators are likely to think they can get away with it, as they are an easy target, no one cares about them. Most disabled people are restricted both economically and geographically to their homes. This can mean that they are often unable to escape their abusers. The other consideration is the use of the internet, which for many has been a positive force but there is evidence of some shocking material about people with learning disability written anonymously. The website 'Coping with Epilepsy' was attacked and hateful massages left.

The role of support services

It is important to understand how this can have life changing effects on the victims. As a professional in such a case, it is important you engage with the existing support networks that victims may have, this makes the experience of reporting hate crime less daunting and may improve reporting. Some police forces have special measures available to help them to give witness accounts; or easy read leaflets. They will be keen to identification early; a person needs support in the reporting stage. If it gets to court there are also special measures in place here, like not having to give evidence in front of the abuser. There is evidence that the increased use of special measures at pre-trial and court stages is yielding results. It is also important to consider a person's health, look for signs of post-traumatic stress disorder (PTSD) for example. Work with the network to get appropriate psychologist or psychiatrist services for the individual or family if required.

A key issue is how society feels it deals with disability. What sort of picture does it have of disability? There has been a significant change in the last 25 years with the closure of the long-stay hospitals for people with learning disabilities. People have moved to live in the community successfully; despite this, the reality is that the majority of the population are ignorant about people and their lives. There is still a great deal of prejudice around. In the summer of 2012, the London Paralympics Games showed very positive images; maybe this is something to build on for professionals.

It is clear that disability organisations have played an important role in publicising hate crimes and demanding more effective responses. The important role for the nursing professional is to see and understand what a hate crime is, and to have a zero tolerance policy. Support people with developing their social networks: the more connected we are to each other, the safer we are. Remember that all that is needed for evil to triumph is for good people to do nothing.

Learning Disability Nursing at a Glance, First Edition. Edited by Bob Gates, Debra Fearns and Jo Welch. © 2015 John Wiley & Sons, Ltd. Published 2015 by John Wiley & Sons, Ltd.
Companion website: www.ataglanceseries.com/nursing/learningdisability

67 Sex and individuals with a learning disability

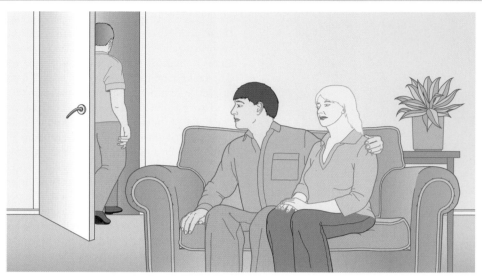

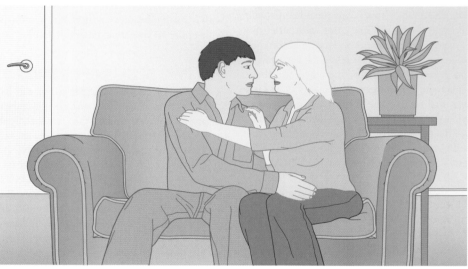

Introduction

In the last 30 years, significant changes have taken place in the way the UK thinks about people with a learning disability, and in its approaches to their needs and those of their families. Society now recognises that adults with a learning disability should be acknowledged as adults whose individual requirements are met without undue separation.

One aspect of adulthood which is taken for granted, is the right to be sexually active. There are two contradictory myths which contribute to people with a learning disability not being automatically included in this right:

• People with a learning disability remain forever childlike and 'innocent', whatever their actual age. As sexual expression within childhood is not usual, it is not seen as appropriate for people with a learning disability to express themselves sexually.

• People with a learning disability have very strong sexual drives and appetites, but very poor self-control, so that they are a danger both to themselves and to other members of society. This is still a recurrent theme that is pervasive in society.

All human are sexual beings. Sexuality is not an optional extra. Everyone has sexual needs, feelings and drives.

People with learning disabilities may need support to manage their needs, feelings and drives to get pleasure and enjoyment from their close personal relationships, and provide them with protection from relationships which may be abusive.

Sex education

Being ignorant in relation to sex education is harmful. For example, not knowing how to behave sexually or the consequences of sexual activity, not knowing the difference between public and private behaviour, not knowing how the body functions in regards to the mechanics of sexual organs. It may lead to people with learning disabilities being unable to say 'no' to touching that make them uncomfortable, and leaves people with a learning disability vulnerable to abuse or exploitation.

Some young people with learning disabilities receive a very negative form of sex education – 'Don't do that, it's not nice', 'Stop touching yourself down there, that's bad!' The effect of them thinking sex is something dirty and shameful can leave long-lasting effects on their self-esteem.

Why people with LD may be more vulnerable to sexual abuse

- They may not possess the social awareness or education to detect or anticipate abusive situations.
- They may be afraid to challenge potentially abusive situations.
- They may be afraid to report abuse after the event, although they recognise what has happened.
- They may have communication difficulties.
- They may feel that nobody will believe them.
- They may have feelings of guilt or shame that prevent them reporting abuse.
- Others may feel that there is nobody to whom they can complain (especially if the abuser is a figure of authority).

Supporting people with learning disabilities

People with a learning disability have a right to a private life and to a life free from abuse. They should not be exposed to greater harm than the general population because of their disability.

- In 2007 The Family Planning Association found that 63% of people with LD wanted to know more about sex and relationships.
- Within care systems, we have to be clear about how people arrive at the decision to say yes (or no) to a sexual relationship and how they go on to negotiate the terms of this relationship.
- We must do everything possible to protect vulnerable people with a learning disability from abuse and respond to abuse when it does take place. The law must be reformed to deter sexual abusers. The existing loopholes must be closed to ensure that abusers are appropriately punished.

Supporting parents/carers

- They may not believe their children will ever marry and have children.
- They may believe their children will need more protection as 'sexual' beings.
- They may have difficulty accepting their 'child' has matured physically or sexually if the 'child' is still behaving immaturely.

Consent/capacity

In 2003 the Sexual Offences Act enshrined in law the view that it is illegal for any sexual touching of a person with a mental disorder which impedes their choices if they:

1 Lack the capacity to agree to be touched.

2 Cannot communicate the choice or agree to be touched because of an inducement, threat or deception.

3 Or cannot give valid consent because the other person with whom they are in relationship is in position of trust with that person.

The Sexual Offences Act 2003 changes the law on rape and sexual assault so that offences include sexual activity with someone who does not have the capacity to consent. The Act makes clear that consent must be freely given. It also provides protection where someone's disability prevents them from communicating whether they want to have sex.

Sexual abuse

We know from our experience that people with learning disabilities are at an increased risk of sexual abuse, and that there is a low conviction rate of those who sexually abuse people with learning disabilities.

Research studies of the sexual abuse of people with a learning disability suggest that at least 1400 adults with a learning disability are likely to be reported as victims of sexual abuse each year.

It has also been proven that disabled people may be up to four times more likely to experience abuse.

Types of sexual offences

- Rape
- Assault by penetration
- Sexual assault
- Inciting sexual activity without consent.

The Act provides specific designated sexual offences. It covers sexual offences including offences against children, adults whose capacity is impaired and familial offences (incest). Newly added offences include 'voyeurism' (a person is observed without consent or knowledge where there is expected privacy). It also requires people convicted of most forms of sexual offence to register their name and address with the local police.

Legislation relevant to protecting people with learning disabilities from sexual offences is as follows:

Sexual Offences Act 2003:

- Section 30: Sexual activity with a person with a mental disorder impeding choice.
- Section 31: Causing or inciting a person, with a mental disorder impeding choice, to engage in sexual activity.
- Section 32: Engaging in sexual activity in the presence of a person with a mental disorder impeding choice.
- Section 33: Causing a person, with a mental disorder impeding choice, to watch a sexual act.
- Section 34: Inducement, threat or deception to procure sexual activity with a person with a mental disorder.
- Section 35: Causing a person with a mental disorder to engage in or agree to engage in sexual activity by inducement, threat or deception.
- Section 36: Engaging in sexual activity in the presence, procured by inducement, threat or deception, of a person with a mental disorder.
- Section 37: Causing a person with a mental disorder to watch a sexual act by inducement, threat or deception.
- Section 38: Care workers: sexual activity with a person with a mental disorder.
- Section 39: Care workers: causing or inciting sexual activity.
- Section 40: Care workers: sexual activity in the presence of a person with a mental disorder.
- Section 41: Care workers: causing a person with a mental disorder to watch a sexual act.

Section 42: **Definition of a care worker**:

- Workers from care/community/voluntary/children's homes.
- Workers from NHS services or independent medical agencies.
- People in regular face-to-face contact with client, regardless of whether they provide physical or mental care.
- Paid or unpaid, full or part-time.

Summary

- The vast majority of individuals with a learning disability develop normally as sexual beings.
- They might need help to understand the bodily and emotional changes that occur as they grow up, but if denied the right to be sexual and to make and break relationships their lives are much poorer.
- Some people with a learning disability may experience abuse if they are not taught about safe, loving relationships.
- People can be referred to specialist support services as well as family planning services.

Spirituality

Spirituality	Spirituality – a broader view
• Spirituality may be religious or non-religious • Everyone has a spirituality • Everyone is unique and so is their spirituality • Everyone is unique and has a spirituality like someone else's spirituality	**Consider the following:** • Relationships • Loneliness • Loss/grief • Space • Spiritual practices

What is spirituality?

Spirituality is more than a word; it is something that can be expressed verbally and through actions. It is an experience that may be heard or seen and that fills the person with awe. It is both a complex and mysterious part of a person's being. Spirituality has been variously defined by many people including nurses, psychologists, theologians and educationalists. It is a word that can be misunderstood as it is very often equated with religion. Every human has a spiritual dimension. It is a multicultural entity and not necessarily placed in a particular religious faith. The last 20 years have seen a renewed interest in spirituality, resulting in it being a popular topic for research as well as a plethora of self-help books on how spirituality can help the individual to develop and have a fulfilled life in a secular world.

Defining spirituality can take a view that assumes particular knowledge and the use of specific language. Taking this narrow approach results in excluding anyone who does not have that special knowledge and is unable to use the specific language required. This would exclude children, children and adults with a learning disability, adults with acquired brain damage, dementia or anyone unfamiliar with the language and culture of the spirituality. Viewing spirituality as having to be learnt and enacted in a particular way is inaccurate. It has been demonstrated that everyone has an awareness of spirituality and that this is apparent in everyday life and is very much a part of how humans relate to one another and the world in which they live.

The consequences of ignoring spirituality

Ignoring spirituality squashes the spiritual life a person has, and in terms of a spiritual faith it can create a view that misunderstands that person's faith, seeing it only as a series of religious targets of knowledge and tasks that have to be achieved, such as reading the Holy Book, prayer and doctrine.

Working alongside a person with learning disability may reveal that the carer has little or no concept of spirituality. This may result in them feeling uncertain or incompetent in meeting a person's particular spiritual needs. The carer may also fear that they are encroaching upon the privacy and therefore the beliefs of the person for whom they are caring. Professional opinion about spirituality may not always be positive. It may be viewed as marginal and not part of any assessment or subsequent intervention.

Spirituality is important

Recent legislation (Equality Act 2010) has included the right to a spiritual life. People cannot be discriminated against on the basis of their religious or non-religious beliefs, including the actions that go with that particular set of beliefs or if they change their beliefs. This is reinforced by the nurses' professional code that holds them accountable for the beliefs that a person in their care holds. The right to a spiritual life requires us to think differently about how the spiritual needs for a person with learning disability will be met. Meeting these needs requires something other than the imposition of another's beliefs, or a response that is merely tokenistic. Everyone has a spirituality which is unique to them, as well as something that is like someone else's spirituality.

Supporting others in their spirituality

Person centred planning empowers people with a learning disability to access services (DoH, 2001). It is an evidence-based process that finds out what the individual wants, the support they would require and how this can be achieved. The physical, social and psychological needs of the person are identified and it is at this point that all those involved in the person centred planning should be listening closely to everything that the person identifies as a want. Spiritual needs require us to think broadly. Spirituality may or may not be a religious experience allied to a particular faith. We need to draw on a variety of resources, using different disciplines such as nursing psychology, theology and education. This grounds us in evidence based practice, rather than purely our own experience.

A broader view of spirituality

How might a person's spirituality manifest its self, whether it is part of a particular religion or not? The individual's spiritual needs may be through relationships; getting to know others through listening and being listened to. Over time this may develop into a number of friendships, which grow in different ways with varying levels of trust and perhaps the realisation that there is a bond of intimacy with some people.

Friendships, as well as being part of various communities, and the involvement that the individual has with these different individuals and groups will, over time, include the loss of people who the person has known. This may be as another person moves away or as they die. There may then be feelings of loneliness. All of which may require support.

Spiritual needs may be to do with a search for meaning and the purpose of life. Wanting to know why I am here, what am I meant to do with my life – through to knowing who I want to share my life with and what that means for the present, the future and what I could become.

The need for space and quiet may be a particular room or a space in part of a room with particular familiar objects. It may be space outside, by the sea or a field or a hill. Here there is the opportunity to think on life, experience peace and comfort and for those with a particular faith to feel able to draw closer to their God.

Learning Disability Nursing at a Glance, First Edition. Edited by Bob Gates, Debra Fearns and Jo Welch. © 2015 John Wiley & Sons, Ltd. Published 2015 by John Wiley & Sons, Ltd.
Companion website: www.ataglanceseries.com/nursing/learningdisability

69 The twenty-first century: Networking for success

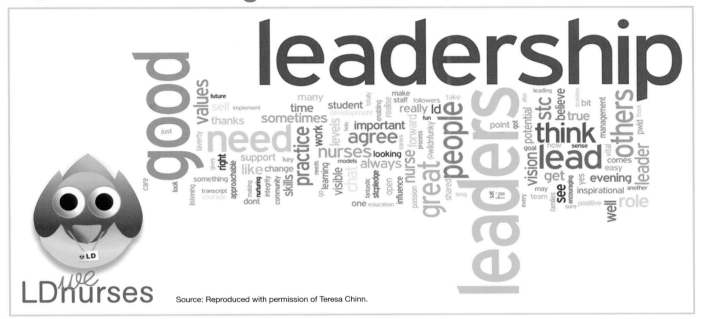

Source: Reproduced with permission of Teresa Chinn.

Twenty-first century LD nursing

The internet is a boundless resource for professional development, and while we use it mostly as a library to view publications and presentations, the relatively recent use of software to enable interaction has significant potential to help users to unpick and understand complex issues.

Learning disability nursing in the twenty-first century remains the smallest field of nursing, and we can be found in a wide variety organisations and a plethora of roles; this can mean limited opportunities for contact with colleagues.

However, learning disability nurses have a long history of making links with other learning disability nurses, locally, regionally and nationally. This enables the sharing of good practice examples and challenges, the asking and answering of questions, and presentation of a unified message to society that people with learning disabilities can live inclusive and valued lives through improved access to the community and the eradication of health inequalities.

The increasingly ubiquitous use of social media can provide learning disability nurses with opportunities to maintain links with like-minded professionals, to consider topics of the day, and reflect on complex subjects. Networks like Twitter, Facebook and LinkedIn, amongst others, provide learning disability nurses with a first step on the road to writing for publication and contributing to the body of knowledge, while also increasing their visibility and that of the profession.

With the online community growing daily and smartphones offering real-time virtual contact, the many possibilities can seem endless. With so many choices, what are the best options?

LinkedIn is a professional networking site. A great way of linking with colleagues around the country and can also be useful when looking for work.

Facebook is a social networking site connecting friends and colleagues alike. There are a number of groups for students and nurses to join, which may be an easy first step into social media. Users can set privacy settings so only friends can see pictures and posts. There are no limits to what you can post, and you can include links to other sites within the post.

Twitter is a real time live conversation (see Figure above). There is no privacy, but there are character limits, 140 characters to make your point can be challenging, but it forces succinctness which can be very refreshing. There is also the opportunity for live twitter chats, which can include anyone who is on twitter at the time. Chats are linked by a hash tag (#) which in effect joins individual tweets and becomes a theme of the conversation.

Blogging is a great way of sharing experiences, thoughts and reflections about all things nursing. It can also be a really useful way to take a second step toward publication.

When we accept the role of nurse, we are bound by the code of conduct set forth by the Nursing and Midwifery Council (NMC). As nurses we have a duty to uphold and maintain the standards and integrity of our profession; as use of social media expands this also extends to our digital footprint. The NMC has produced guidelines on the safe use of social media and should always be considered by all nurses. In addition to this, local policies may be in place within your organisation. It is important to familiarise yourself with such guidance to ensure that online activities maintain these standards.

Learning Disability Nursing at a Glance, First Edition. Edited by Bob Gates, Debra Fearns and Jo Welch. © 2015 John Wiley & Sons, Ltd. Published 2015 by John Wiley & Sons, Ltd.
Companion website: www.ataglanceseries.com/nursing/learningdisability

The value of social media as a networking, professional and educational tool should not be disregarded. Understanding appropriate and acceptable online behaviours, we should reflect on what we would consider appropriate and acceptable behaviours in the 'real world'; politeness, courtesy and respect are key to maintaining professional standards both in the real and virtual worlds.

In 2012, four learning disability nurses were involved in a Twitter chat via @wenurses, throughout the chat it became apparent that they were the only self-identifying LD nurses contributing. After the chat the four nurses had a virtual conversation and agreed to set up a fortnightly twitter chat for anyone involved in learning disability healthcare. Twitter chats appealed to this group as this media had no respect for organisational boundaries or hierarchies, and as such enabled a truly democratic space for debate and discussion. It was also believed that this would be an ideal forum to consider how the values and recommendations of Strengthening the Commitment are reflected in day-to-day practice.

Topics for fortnightly discussions are suggested by participants and scheduled by the team. The chat is then announced on the designated Facebook page and also on WeNurses.com with referenced pre-chat reading material that has been produced by those who suggested the topic in collaboration with the team.

After each discussion the transcript is published on WeNurses. This is closely followed by a blog that draws on the themes of chat, offering further analysis, interpretation and creative ways of sharing the discussion (see Figure above).

The chats often cross fields of practice encouraging collaboration with professionals involved in other forums, such as mental health, adult and child health trained nurses, psychologists, behavioural analysts, occupational therapists, speech and language therapists, parents/carers and people with learning disabilities. Since its inception the chats – previously known as @ldnursechat, and now as @WeLDnurses – have gathered over 1300 followers; have held over 24 chats with over 200 people participating, and have contributed to the English Chief Nursing Officer's consultation Compassion in Practice.

Summary

- There are opportunities in the twenty-first century for learning disability nurses to promote and develop practice using the technologies that most of us use for social contact and swiftly identify electronic methods for developing their own practice and that of others.
- This increases our visibility and that of our profession and as such prompts us to consider how we communicate with each other in front of a global audience.
- @WeLDnurses provides a good example of how social media can be harnessed to share innovation and inspiration.

Further reading and resources

Part 1: Introduction to learning disability nursing

Aldridge, J. (2004) Intellectual disability nursing: a model for practice. In: J. Turnbull (ed.) *Learning Disability Nursing*. Blackwell Publishing: Oxford, pp. 169–187.

Department of Health (2001) *Valuing People: A New Strategy for Learning Disability for the 21st Century*. DoH: London.

Department of Health (2007) *Good Practice in Learning Disability Nursing*. DoH: London.

Department of Health (2009) *Valuing People Now: A New Three Year Strategy for People with Learning Disabilities*. DoH: London.

Department of Health (2013) *Mid Staffordshire NHS Foundation Trust Public Inquiry: Government Response*. http://francisresponse. dh.gov.uk/values-and-standards/ [Accessed October 2014].

Francis, R. (2013) *Report of the Mid Staffordshire NHS Foundation Trust Public Inquiry*. The Stationery Office: England.

Gates, B. (ed.) (1997) Understanding learning disability. In: *Learning Disabilities*, 3rd edn. Churchill Livingstone: Edinburgh, pp. 16–17.

Gates, B. (2006) *Care Planning and Care Delivery in Intellectual Disability Nursing*. Blackwell Science: London.

Nursing and Midwifery Council (2010) *Standards for Pre-registration Nursing Education*. NMC: London.

Orem, D. E. (1991) *Nursing: Concepts of Practice*. Mosby: St Louis, MO.

Roper, N., Logan, W. & Tierney, A. (2002) *The Elements of Nursing*, 4th edn. Churchill Livingstone: Edinburgh.

Scottish Government (2013) *Modernising Learning Disabilities Nursing Review*. http://www.rcn.org.uk/__data/assets/pdf_ file/0004/521158/national_framework_for_prereg_ld_nursing_ field_progs.pdf [Accessed May 2013].

UK Chief Nursing Officers (2012) *Strengthening the Commitment. The Report of the UK Modernising Learning Disabilities Nursing Review*. Scottish Government: Edinburgh.

Part 2: Exploration of learning disability

American Association of Intellectual and Developmental Disability (2010). *Intellectual Disability: Definition, Classification, and Systems of Supports*, 11th edn. AAIDD: Washington.

Contact A Family: http://www.cafamily.org.uk/ [Accessed May 2013].

Department of Health: https://www.gov.uk/government/ organisations/department-of-health [Accessed May 2014].

Gates, B. (ed.) (1997) Understanding learning disability. In: *Learning Disabilities*, 3rd edn. Churchill Livingstone: Edinburgh, pp. 16–17.

Klotz, J. (2004) Sociocultural study of intellectual disability: moving beyond labelling and social constructionist perspectives. *British Journal of Learning Disabilities* 32: 93–4.

MENCAP: http://www.mencap.org.uk/all-about-learning-disability [Accessed May 2014].

Part 3: Childhood development

Brock, A., Dodds, S., Jarvis, P., & Olusoga, Y. (2008) *Perspectives on Play, Learning for Life*. Pearson; London.

Cole, K. (2001) *Supervision: The Theory and Practice of First-line Management*. Pearson Education: Frenchs Forest, Australia.

Cole, C., Pointu, A., Wellsted, D. M., & Angus-Leppan, H. A. (2010) A pilot study of the epilepsy risk awareness checklist (ERAC) in people with epilepsy and learning disabilities. *Seizure - European Journal of Epilepsy* 19: 592–596.

Meggitt, C. (2007) *Child Development: An Illustrated Guide, Birth to 16 Years*, 3rd edn. Heinemann: London.

Mehrabian, A. (1971) *Silent Messages*. Wadsworth: Belmont, CA, pp. 44–45.

NHS Start 4 Life: http://www.nhs.uk/Tools/Pages/birthtofive. aspx#close [Accessed May 2014].

UK Government (2012) *Draft Legislation on Reform of Provision for Children and Young People with Special Educational Needs*. http:// www.officialdocuments.gov.uk/document/cm84/8438/8438.pdf [Accessed May 2014].

UK Government (2014) *Support for Children and Young People*. http://www.education.gov.uk/schools/pupilsupport/sen [Accessed May 2014].

Part 4: Adolescence

American Psychiatric Association (2013) *Diagnostic and Statistical Manual of Mental Disorders*, 5th edn (DSM-5). American Psychiatric Association: Washington, DC.

Aylott, J. (2011) *The Autism Act 2009: Developing Specialist Skills in Autism Practice*. http://rcnpublishing.com/userimages/ ContentEditor/1373364280087/Autism-booklet-2011.pdf [Accessed May 2014].

Bailey, J. (2005) *Sex Puberty and All That Stuff*. Franklin Watts: Australia.

Department of Health (1998) *Teenage Pregnancy Strategy*. DoH: London.

Department of Health (2004) *Every Child Matters - A Change for Children*. DoH: London.

NSPCC (2010) *Research Briefing: School Bullying*. http://www.nspcc. org.uk/inform/research/briefings/school_bullying_pdf_wdf73502. pdf [Accessed May 2014].

Public Health England: http://www.improvinghealthandlives.org.uk/ [Accessed May 2014].

The Road Ahead: Literature Review. http://www.scie.org.uk/ publications/tra/files/literature.pdf [Accessed May 2014].

UK Government (2003) Sexual Offences Act. http://www.legislation. gov.uk/ukpga/2003/42 [Accessed May 2014].

UK Government (2009) Autism Act. http://www.legislation.gov.uk/ ukpga/2009/15/contents [Accessed May 2014].

Part 5: Adults with a learning disability

Abudarham, S. & Hurd, A. (2002) *Management of Communication Needs: In People with Learning Disability*. Whurr Publishers: London.

Emerson, E. & Baines, S. (2010) *Health Inequalities & People with Learning Disabilities in the UK: 2010*. http://www. improvinghealthandlives.org.uk/uploads/doc/vid_7479_ IHaL2010-3HealthInequality2010.pdf [Accessed May 2014].

Hannah, N., Black, M., Sander, J. et al. (2002) *National Sentinel Audit into Epilepsy-Related Death: Epilepsy – Death in the Shadows*. HMS: London.

Learning Disability Nursing at a Glance, First Edition. Edited by Bob Gates, Debra Fearns and Jo Welch. © 2015 John Wiley & Sons, Ltd. Published 2015 by John Wiley & Sons, Ltd.
Companion website: www.ataglanceseries.com/nursing/learningdisability

IASSID (2001) Clinical guidelines for the management of epilepsy in adults with an intellectual disability. *Seizure* 10: 401–409.

NICE (2011) *Autism Diagnosis in Children and Young People: Recognition, Referral and Diagnosis of Children and Young People on the Autism Spectrum.* http://guidance.nice.org.uk/CG128 [Accessed May 2014].

NICE (2012) *The Epilepsies: The Diagnosis and Management of the Epilepsies in Adults and Children in Primary and Secondary Care.* http://www.nice.org.uk/guidance/cg137 [Accessed May 2014].

Part 6: People with learning disability and additional mental health needs

Chaplin, R. (2004*) General psychiatric services for adults with intellectual disabilities and mental illness. Journal of Intellectual Disability Research 48: 1, 1–10.

Diagnosis of personality disorders in learning disability (2013) DoH (2011) *Positive Practice, Positive Outcomes: A Handbook for Professionals in the Criminal Justice System working with Offenders with Learning Disabilities.* DoH: London.

Emerson, E. (2001) *Challenging Behaviour: Analysis and intervention in people with severe intellectual disabilities,* 2nd edn. Cambridge University Press: Cambridge, p3.

La Vigna, G.W. & Willis, T. J. (2005) Episodic Severity: an overlooked dependent variable in the application of behavior analysis to challenging behavior. *Journal of Positive Behavior Interventions* 7: 47–54.

Moss, S., Prosser, H., Costello, H. et al. (1998) Reliability and validity of the PAS ADD Checklist for Reliability and validity of the PAS ADD Checklist for detecting psychiatric disorders in adults with intellectual detecting psychiatric disorders in adults with intellectual disability. *Journal of Intellectual Disability Research* 42: 173–183.

NICE Guidance: Challenging Behaviour: http://guidance.nice.org.uk/CG/Wave0/654 [Accessed May 2014].

Nirje, B. (1969) The normalization principle and its human management implications. In: R. Kugel and W. Wolfensberger (eds.) *Changing Patterns in Residential Services for the Mentally Retarded.* President's Committee on Mental Retardation: Washington, DC, pp. 179–195.

O'Brien, J. & Tyne, A. (1981) *The Principle of Normalisation : A Foundation for Effective Services.* Campaign for Mental Handicapped People: London.

Priest, H. & Gibbs, M. (2004) *Mental Health for People with Learning Disabilities.* Churchill Livingstone: Edinburgh, p7.

PRT (2007) *No One Knows: Offenders with Learning Difficulties and Learning Disabilities.* http://www.prisonreformtrust.org.uk/uploads/documents/NOKNL.pdf [Accessed March 2014].

Raghavan, R., Marshall, M., Lockwood, A. & Duggan, L. (2004) Assessing the needs of people with learning disabilities and mental illness: development of the Learning Disability version of the Cardinal Needs Schedule. *Journal of Intellectual Disability Research* 48(1):25–36

The Rt Hon Lord Bradley (2009) *Lord Bradley's Review of People with Mental Health Problems and Learning Disabilities in the Criminal Justice System.* DoH: London

Royal College of Nursing (2013) *Provision of Mental Health Care for Adults who have a Learning Disability.* RCN: London.

Royal College of Psychiatrists (2001) *DC-LD Diagnostic Criteria for Psychiatric Disorders for Use with Adults with Learning Disabilities/Mental Retardation.* Gaskell: London.

Wolfensberger, W. (1972) *The Principle of Normalization in Human Services.* National Institute on Mental Retardation: Toronto.

Xenitidis, K., Thornicroft, G., Leese, M. et al. (2000) Reliability and validity of the CANDID - a needs assessment instrument for adults with learning disabilities and mental health problems. *British Journal of Psychiatry* 176: 473–478

Part 7: Vulnerable adults with a learning disability

British Institute of Human Rights: http://www.bihr.org.uk/resources/useful-links [Accessed May 2014].

Department for Constitutional Affairs (2007) *Making Decisions: A Guide for People Working in Health and Social Care.* Booklet 3 in a series of 5. Department for Constitutional Affairs: London.

The Equality Authority (2010) *Your Equal Status Rights Explained: Guide to the Equal Status Acts 2000–2008.* https://www.tcd.ie/equality/assets/pdf/equal-status-actguidebook.pdf [Accessed May 2014].

House of Lords and House of Commons Joint Report (2007–2008) *A Life Like Any Other? Human Rights of Adults with Learning Disabilities.* http://www.publications.parliament.uk/pa/jt200708/jtselect/jtrights/40/40i.pdf [Accessed May 2014].

Jepson, M. (2008) Who decides? Using the Mental Capacity Act to support people. *Learning Disability Today* 8(1): 22–27.

Joyce, T. (2007) *Best Interests: Guidance on Determining the Best Interests of Adults who Lack the Capacity to Make a Decision (or Decisions) for Themselves.* British Psychology Society: Leicester.

Office of the Public Guardian (2009) *Making Decisions: A Guide for Family, Friends and Other Unpaid Carers. Mental Capacity Implementation Programme.* OPG: England.

Roach, M.S. (2002) *Caring, the Human Mode of Being: A Blueprint for the Health Professions* (2nd revised edn). Canadian Hospital Association Press: Ottawa, Ontario, p66.

Scottish Government (2010) The Equality Act. http://www.legislation.gov.uk/ssi/2012/162/contents/made

Scottish Government (2012) *Strengthening the Commitment: The Report of the UK Modernising Learning Disabilities Nursing Review.* Scottish Government: Edinburgh.

Tschudin, V. (ed) (1993) *Nurses and patients.* Scutari Press: Middlesex, pp 9–15.

Tschudin, V. (2003) *Ethics in Nursing: The Caring Relationship.* Butterworth-Heinemann: London.

Williams, V., Jepson, M., Tarleton, B. et al. (2008) *Listen to what I want: The potential impact of the Mental Capacity Act (2005) on major life decisions by people with learning disabilities.* Social Care Institute for Excellence: Bristol.

UK Government (2005) Mental Capacity Act. http://www.legislation.gov.uk/ukpga/2005/9/contents [Accessed May 2014].

UK Government (2007) Mental Health Act. http://www.legislation.gov.uk/ukpga/2007/12/contents [Accessed May 2014].

UK Government (2008) Mental Health Act Code of Practice. http://www.lbhf.gov.uk/Images/Code%20of%20practice%201983%20rev%202008%20dh_087073%5B1%5D_tcm21-145032.pdf [Accessed May 2014].

UK Government (2010) Equality Act. http://www.legislation.gov.uk/ukpga/2010/15/contents [Accessed May 2014].

Part 8: Biophysical aspects of learning disability nursing

Brown, M., MacArthur, J., McKechanie, A. et al. (2011) Learning disability liaison nursing services in South-East Scotland: a mixed-methods impact and outcome study. *Journal of Intellectual Ability Research* 56(12): 1161–74.

Brown, H., Burns, S. & Flynn, M. (2005) *Dying Matters: A Workbook on Caring for People with Learning Disabilities who are Terminally Ill.* Mental Health Foundation: London.

Department of Health (2009) *Health Action Planning and Health Facilitation for People with Learning Disabilities; Good Practice Guide.* DoH: London.

Department of Health (2012) *Transforming Care: A National Response to Winterbourne View Hospital.* DoH: London.

Department of Health, Social Services and Public Safety (2012) *Fit and Well 2012–2022: A 10 Year Public Health and Tackling Health Inequalities Strategic Framework*. DHSSPS: Belfast.

Department of Health, Social Services and Public Safety (2012) *Learning Disability Service Framework*. DHSSPS: Belfast.

Emerson, E. & Hatton, C. (2008) *People with Learning Disabilities in England*. CeDR Research Report 2008:1. CEDR: Lancaster, England, p5.

Gates, R. (2009) *The Valued People Project: Report of a Strategic Review of Educational Commissioning and Workforce Planning in Learning Disabilities*. NHS Education South Central: England, p52.

Gates, R. (2009). Nursing patients with a learning disability. In G. Castledine & A. Close (eds.) *Oxford Handbook of Adult Nursing*. OUP: England, pp 973–82.

Guideline and Audit Information Network (2010) *Improving the quality experience of people with a Learning Disability in General Hospital Settings*. GAIN: Belfast.

Howatson, J. (2005) Health action plans for people with learning disabilities. *Nursing Standard* 19(43): 51–57.

Health Needs Assessment Report: People with Learning Disabilities in Scotland (2004) http://www.gla.ac.uk/media/media_63872_en.pdf [Accessed May 2014].

Health Inequalities and People with Learning Disabilities (2010) http://www.improvinghealthandlives.org.uk/uploads/doc/vid_7479_IHaL2010-3HealthInequality2010.pdf [Accessed May 2014].

Health Inequalities and People with Learning Disabilities in the UK (2010) *Implications and Actions for Commissioners*. http://www.ndti.org.uk/uploads/files/IHAL201001_Health_Inequalities4_(3).pdf [Accessed May 2014].

Health Checks for People with Learning Disabilities: A Systematic Review of Evidence. http://www.improvinghealthandlives.org.uk/uploads/doc/vid_7646_IHAL2010-04HealthChecksSystemticReview.pdf [Accessed May 2014].

Improving Health and Lives Learning Disabilities Observatory (2012) *Confidential Inquiry into Premature Death of People with Learning Disabilities*. IHAL: Bristol.

Improving the Health and Wellbeing of People with Learning Disabilities: An Evidence-Based Commissioning Guide for Clinical Commissioning Groups (CCGs) (2012). http://www.rcgp.org.uk/revalidation-and-cpd/centreforcommissioning/~/media/Files/CIRC/LD%20Commissioning/RCGP%20LD%20Commissioning%20Guide%20v1%200%202012%2009%2024%20FINAL%20pdf.ashx [Accessed May 2014].

Kerr, D. (2007) *Understanding Learning Disability and Dementia: Developing Effective Interventions*. Kingsley: London.

McCaffery, M. (1972) *Nursing Management of the Patient in Pain*. JB Lippincott: Philadelphia, p8.

Mencap (2012) *Death by Indifference: 74 Deaths and Counting. A Progress Report Five Years On*. Mencap: London.

Michael, J. (2008) *Healthcare For All: Report of the Independent Inquiry into Access to Healthcare for People with Learning Disabilities*. www.iahpld.org.uk [Accessed May 2014].

National Patients Safety Agency (2004) *Understanding the Patient Safety Issues for People with Learning Disabilities*. NPSA: London.

NHS Scotland (2008) *Improving General Hospital Care for People with Learning Disabilities in Scotland*. http://a2anetwork.co.uk/wp-content/uploads/2009/06/Michael-Brown-Improving-general-hospital-care-for-pwld.pdf [Accessed May 2014].

Parliamentary and Public Health Service Ombudsmen (2009) *Six Lives: The Provision of Public Services to People with Learning Disabilities*. The Stationery Office: London.

Royal College of Nursing (2013) *Meeting the Health Needs of People with Learning Disabilities*. http://www.rcn.org.uk/__data/assets/pdf_file/0004/78691/003024.pdf [Accessed May 2014].

Royal College of Nursing (2013) *Dignity in Health Care for People with Learning Disabilities*. RCN: London.

Part 9: Older people with learning disability

Centre for Research on Families (2006) *Best Practice in Learning Disability and Dementia: Getting Service User Views*. https://www.era.lib.ed.ac.uk/bitstream/1842/2781/1/rb28.pdf [Accessed May 2014].

Joseph Rowntree Foundation (2012) *Perspectives on Ageing with a Learning Disability*. http://www.jrf.org.uk/sites/files/jrf/ageing-and-learning-disability-summary.pdf [Accessed May 2014].

McCarron, M., Swinburne, J., Burke, E. et al. (2011) *Growing Older with an Intellectual Disability in Ireland 2011: First Results from The Intellectual Disability Supplement of The Irish Longitudinal Study on Ageing*. http://www.hrb.ie/uploads/media/Growing_Older_with_an_Intellectual_Disability_in_Ireland_2011.pdf [Accessed May 2014].

NHS End of Life Care (2011) *The Route to Success in End of Life Care - Achieving Quality for People with Learning Disabilities*. http://www.nhsiq.nhs.uk/resource-search/publications/eolc-rts-learning-disabilities.aspx [Accessed May 2014].

NICE NHS Dementia guidelines (2006) *Supporting People with Dementia and their Carers in Health and Social Care*. http://www.nice.org.uk/nicemedia/pdf/cg042niceguideline.pdf [Accessed May 2014].

Royal College of Psychiatrists (2009) *Dementia and People with Learning Disabilities: Guidance on the Assessment, Diagnosis, Treatment and Support of People with Learning Disabilities who Develop Dementia*. http://www.rcpsych.ac.uk/files/pdfversion/cr155.pdf [Accessed May 2014].

Part 10: Medication

Bhaumik, S. & Branford, D. (2005) *The Frith Prescribing Guidelines for Adults with Learning Disability*. Taylor and Francis: London and New York.

National Patient Safety Agency (2009) *Safety in Doses: Improving the Use of Medicines in the NHS*. NPSA: London.

National Prescribing Centre (2007) *A Competency Framework for Shared Decision Making with Patients, Achieving Concordance for Taking Medicines*, 1st edn. NPC Plus: England.

Nursing and Midwifery Council (2006) *Standards of Proficiency for Nurse and Midwife Prescribers*. NMC Publications: London.

Nursing and Midwifery Council (2010) *Standards for Medicines Management*. NMC Publications: London.

Part 11: The learning disability nurse

Castle, M. (2012) *Learning Disability Acute Liaison Service - Is it Effective?* (PowerPoint slides) Lecture handouts, Hertfordshire University, 21st November 2012.

Castle, A. (2012) Role of liaison nurses in improving communication. *Learning Disability Practice* 15(9): 16–190.

Department of Health (2009) *Health Action Planning and Health Facilitation for People with Learning Disabilities: Good Practice Guide*. DoH: London.

Emerson, E. & Hatton, C. (2008) *People with Learning Disabilities in England*. CeDR Research Report 2008:1. CEDR: Lancaster, England, p5.

Gates, R. (2009) *The Valued People Project: Report of a Strategic Review of Educational Commissioning and Workforce Planning in Learning Disabilities*. NHS Education South Central: Newbury, p52.

Loucks, N. (2007) *No One Knows: Offenders with Learning Difficulties and Learning Disabilities*. Prison Reform Trust: London.

Talbot, J. (2008) *No One Knows: Prisoners' Voices*. Prison Reform Trust: London.

Part 12: Inclusion

Atkinson, D. (1999) *Advocacy: A Review*. Pavilion/Joseph Rowntree Foundation: Brighton.

Brandon, D. (1995) *Advocacy-Power to People with Disabilities*. Venture Press/BASW: Birmingham.

Cambridge, P. & Carnaby, S. (eds) (2005) *Person Centred Planning and Care Management with People with Learning Disabilities*. Kingsley: London.

College of Occupational Therapists (2007*) Work Matter: Vocational Navigation for Occupational Therapy Staff*. DoH: London, p9.

Crawley, B. (1988) *The Growing Voice: A survey of Self-Advocacy Groups in Adult Training Centres and Hospitals*. London: CMH.

Department of Health (2007) *A Jigsaw of Services: Inspection of services to support disabled adults in their parenting role*. The Social Services Inspectorate: London.

Dimond, B. (2007) Mental capacity and decision-making: defining capacity. *British Journal of Nursing* 16(18): pp1138–1139.

Emerson, E. & Hatton, C. (2008) *People with Learning Disabilities in England*. CeDR Research Report 2008:1. CEDR: Lancaster, England.

Inclusion Ireland: A Guide to Disability Law and Policy in Ireland. http://www.inclusionireland.ie/sites/default/files/documents/information_pack-final.pdf [Accessed May 2014].

Jenkins, R. & Northway, R. (2002) Advocacy and the learning disability nurse. *British Journal of Learning Disabilities* 30(1): 8–12.

Narayanasamy, A. (2006) *Spiritual Care and Transcultural Care Research*. Quay: London.

Submission to Mental Capacity Law in Ireland (2011) http://mentalhealthreform.ie/docs/MentalHealthReformSubmissionOnCapacityLegislation2012.pdf [Accessed May 2014].

The Stephen Lawrence Inquiry (1999) *The Stephen Lawrence Inquiry: Report of an Inquiry by Sir William Macpherson of Kluny*. Stationary Office: London, p49, para 6.34.

UK Government (2005) Mental Capacity Act.

UKCC (1998) *Guidelines for Mental Health and Learning Disabilities Nursing*. UKCC: London.

Winstow, R., & Schneifer, J. (2003) Users views on supported employment and social inclusion: a qualitative study of 30 people in work. *British Journal of Learning Disabilities* 31(4): 166–173.

Index

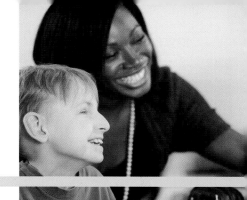

6Cs 6
acute healthcare facilitator 125
adolescence 39–47
  bullying 42–43
  child and adolescent mental
    health services 44–45
  family transitions 47
  individual transitions 47
  psychological distress 44–45
  puberty 40–41
  roles of learning disability
    nurse 41, 47
  transitions 46–47
adult placements 139
adults with learning
    disability 49–61
  biophysical aspects 87, 94–97
  communication skills 52–53
  complex health needs 51
  epilepsy 58–61
  living with autistic spectrum
    conditions 56–57
  national policies 51
  person-centred care 51
  sensory impairment 54–55
  vulnerable adults 73–83
  working with 50–51
  see also older people
advocacy 122, 148–149
affect assessment 109
age discrimination 79
alcohol-related birth defects
    (ARBDs) 13
Alzheimer's disease 87, 96–97,
    106–107
amniocentesis 22
Angelman syndrome 17
ante-natal care 143
antidepressant drugs 45,
    112–113
antiepileptic drugs
    (AEDs) 114–115
antipsychotic drugs 45, 112–113
anxiety disorders 86–87, 89, 113
assessment and treatment (A&T)
    LD nurse 2–3, 128–129
Assessment of Motor and
    Process skills (AMPs) 97
astigmatism 55

attention 28–29
atypical antipsychotics 112–113
autistic spectrum conditions
    (ASC) 34–35, 56–57
autonomy 45, 82–83
autosomal dominant/recessive
    inheritance 23

behavioural phenotypes 11
behavioural presentation 109
beneficence 82–83
best interests 74
bilingualism 29
biophysical aspects 85–101
    common health issues 86–89
    dementia in people with
      Down's syndrome 87,
      96–97
    Health Action
      Planning 90–91
    learning disabilities 86–87
    mental health issues 86–89
    pain assessment and
      recognition 92–93
    palliative and end-of-life
      care 94–95
    postural care 100–101
    role of learning disability
      nurse 91, 95, 99
    sexual health issues 98–99
bio-psychosocial model of
    ageing 104
birth asphyxia 18–19
birth injury 18–19
blogging 155–156
bloodspot screen 22
body shape distortion
    100–101
Bradley Report (2009) 131
brain damage 51
British National Formulary
    (BNF) 117
bullying 42–43, 151

cancer 86, 89
capacity 83, 149, 153
capsules 119
care 6
care planning 3, 147

care programme approach
    (CPA) 69
challenging behaviour
    (CB) 64–65
Chicken pox 13, 26–27
child abuse and neglect 36–37
child and adolescent mental
    health (CAMH)
    services 44–45
childhood development 21–37
    adolescence 40–41
    changes from SEN Code of
      Practice (2001) 33
    common childhood
      diseases 26–27
    definition of learning
      difficulties 32–33
    developing
      communication 28–31
    developmental
      milestones 24–25
    education 32–33
    identifying special educational
      needs 33
    learning through play 30–31
    legislation and statutory
      guidance 33
    safeguarding children 36–37
    screening and genetic
      testing 22–23
    screening for autistic
      spectrum conditions 34–35
Children Act (2004) 37
chorionic villus sampling 22
chromosomal disorders
    14–15, 23
chronic pain 93
citizen advocacy 148–149
clozapine 113
coeliac disease 86
cognition assessment 109
Cognitive Behaviour Therapy
    (CBT) 45
collective advocacy 148–149
commitment 6, 83, 122
communication
    6Cs 6
    adults with learning
      disability 52–53

assessment and treatment
    learning disability
    nurse 129
childhood
    development 28–31
community learning disability
    nurse 122
inclusion 145, 146–147
NMC standards 4–5
older people 109
palliative and end-of-life
    care 95
service user's
    perspective 146–147
vulnerable adults 75
communication chain 52
community 135, 139
community learning disability
    nurse 2, 122–123
Community Teams 104
compassion 6, 83
competence 6, 83
conductive hearing loss 55
confidence 83
congenital anomaly screen 22
congenital hypothyroidism 23
conscience 83
consent 83, 153
constipation 86, 88–89
coronary heart disease
    (CHD) 86, 88–89
courage 6
creativity 122
Cri-du-chat syndrome 16–17
crime prosecution service
    (CPS) 71
criminal justice system 130–131
cultural sensitivity 140
cystic fibrosis (CF) 23

decision making
    ethics 82–83
    NMC standards 4–5
    nurse prescribing 116
    vulnerable adults 74–75,
      82–83
dementia 87, 96–97, 106–107
dental hygiene 86, 88
depression 87, 89, 107, 113

Learning Disability Nursing at a Glance, First Edition. Edited by Bob Gates, Debra Fearns and Jo Welch. © 2015 John Wiley & Sons, Ltd. Published 2015 by John Wiley & Sons, Ltd.
Companion website: www.ataglanceseries.com/nursing/learningdisability

development *see* childhood development
diabetes 86, 87
Diagnostic and Statistical Manual of Mental Disorders (DSM) 34–35, 67, 69
Diagnostic criteria for psychiatric disorders for people with Learning Disabilities (DC-LD) 109
diagnostic overshadowing 93
Dialectical Behaviour Therapy (DBT) 45
diazepam 60–61
dignity 95
Disability Discrimination Act (DDA) 78–79, 136, 137
Disability Employment Advisors (DEA) 137
Down's syndrome 14–15
   biophysical aspects 87, 96–97
   dementia 87, 96–97
   screening and genetic testing 22–23
drug calculations 118–119

early onset dementia 97
ear wax 55
education
   changes from SEN Code of Practice 33
   childhood development 32–33
   definition of learning difficulties 32–33
   ethnic minorities 141
   identifying special educational needs 33
   inclusion 141, 143
   legislation and statutory guidance 33
   parents with a learning disability 143
   sexual health issues 98
Edward's syndrome 14–15
emergency care 61
emotional abuse 36–37
emotions 40
empathy 122
employment
   advantages for employers 137
   barriers to 136
   historical development 136
   inclusion 134, 136–137
   reasonable adjustments 137
   support types 136
   types of 136
   vulnerable adults 79
end-of-life care 94–95
epilepsy 58–61
   assessment and diagnosis 58–59
   biophysical aspects 86, 88–89

differential diagnosis 58
   management of 60–61
   medications 59, 114–115
Equality Act (2010) 78–79
ethics 82–83
ethnic minorities 140–141
European Convention of Human Rights (ECHR) 77
Every Child Matters (2003) 37
expressive language 29, 52–53

family
   adolescence 47
   family support 2
   inclusion 134–135, 139, 144–145, 153
   palliative and end-of-life care 95
   vulnerable adults 75
feeding problems 87
first aid management 61
foetal alcohol syndrome (FASDs) 13, 19
foetal varicella syndrome (FVS) 13
folic acid 13
fostering 139
Fragile X 15

games 31
gastro-intestinal problems 86, 88–89
gastro-oesophageal reflux disease (GORD) 86
genetic disorders 16–17
genetic testing 22–23
German measles 13, 26–27
Glasgow Anxiety Scale (GAS) 108–109
Glasgow Depression Scale (GDS) 108–109
guardianship 80

hand, foot and mouth disease 26–27
hate crime 151
Health Action Planning (HAP) 51, 90–91, 127
healthcare facilitator 124–125
health facilitator 126–127
health inequalities 104–105, 141
health liaison nurse 126–127, 147
health passports 150
health promotion and facilitation 123
hearing impairments 54–55, 87–89
hearing screen 22
Helicobacter pylori 86
holistic nursing 3, 122
home ownership 139
homophobia 42

hospital liaison nurse 126–127, 147
hospital orders 80
hospital type accommodation 138–139
hostels 138–139
housing 138–139
human rights 76–77, 83
Human Rights Act (1998) 77
hypermetropia 54–55
hypothyroidism 87
hypoxic ischaemic encephalopathy (HIE) 18–19

imaginary play 31
impetigo 26–27
inclusion 133–156
   advocacy 148–149
   employment 134, 136–137
   ethnic minorities 140–141
   family 134–135, 139, 144–145, 153
   hate crime 151
   health passports 150
   health, social care and education inequalities 141
   housing and leisure 134, 138–139
   networking and social media 155–156
   older people 105
   parents with a learning disability 142–143
   person-centred planning 134–135, 145
   service user's perspective 146–147
   sex 152–153
   spirituality 154
Independent Mental Capacity Advocates (IMCA) 74–75, 148–149
Independent Mental Health Advocates (IMHA) 81
industrial therapy 136
injections 119
innovation 122
inpatient roles 2–3
insight assessment 109
institutional racism 141
intentional communities 139
interdisciplinary teams 2–3
interests 134, 138–139
International Classification of Disease (ICD-10) 67, 69
interpersonal skills *see* communication and interpersonal skills
intracranial haemorrhage (ICH) 18–19
intrauterine infections 18–19
intrauterine toxins 18–19

job coaching 136
Joint Committee on Human Rights (JCHR) 77
justice 82–83

Klinefelter's syndrome 14–15

language development 28–29
leadership skills 2, 4–5
Learning Difficulty Assessment (LDA) 32–33
learning disability (LD)
   additional needs 11
   behavioural phenotypes 11
   biophysical aspects 86–87
   causes of 12–19
   chromosomal disorders 14–15
   concepts and definitions 10–11
   coping with everyday life 10–11
   degrees of learning disability 11
   during and shortly after birth 13, 18–19
   genetic disorders 16–17
   intellectual profile 10
   maternal factors 12–13, 18–19
   non-verbal abilities 10
   theoretical perspectives 11
   verbal abilities 10
leisure activities 134, 138–139
life stories 107
lifestyle 59, 86–87
liquid medications 119
listening 28–29, 52
lycra suits 101

management skills 2, 4–5
maternal factors 12–13, 18–19
measles 26–27
measles, mumps and rubella (MMR) vaccine 27
medication
   antidepressant and antipsychotic drugs 45, 112–113
   antiepileptic drugs 114–115
   drug calculations 118–119
   nurse prescribing 116–117
   see also individual drugs
medium-chain acylcarnitine deficiency (MCAD) 23
memories 107
Mental Capacity Act (MCA) 74–75, 149
Mental Health Act (1983) 80–81
Mental Health Act (2007) 67, 149

mental health needs 63–71
  adolescence 44–45
  approaches to care and
    management 64–71
  assessment and
    diagnosis 64–71
  biophysical aspects 86–89
  common conditions 66–67
  managing challenging
    behaviour 64–65
  offenders with a learning
    disability 70–71
  older people 104, 106–109
  personality disorder 68–69
  vulnerable adults 80
Mental State Examination
  (MSE) 108–109
midazolam 60–61
Molluscum contagiosum 26–27
mood assessment 109
mumps 26–27
myopia 54–55

National Health Service (NHS)
  Outcomes Framework 150
National Patient Safety Agency
  (NPSA) 119
neglect 36–37
neonatal sepsis 18–19
networking 155–156
neural tube defects 13
Neuropsychological Assessment
  of Dementia on Intellectual
  Disabilities (NAID) 97
newborn screens 22–23
non-maleficence 82–83
non-medical prescribing
  (NMP) 116–117
non-verbal abilities 10
nurse prescribing 116–117
Nursing and Midwifery Council
  (NMC) standards 4–5, 7,
  117, 119
nursing models 3
nursing principles
  6Cs 6
  causes of learning
    disability 18–19
  NMC standards 4–5, 7
  roles of learning disability
    nurses 2–3
  student nurses 7

obesity 87–89
objects of reference 53
offenders with a learning
  disability 70–71, 80
older people 103–109
  biophysical aspects 87, 94–97
  bio-psychosocial model of
    ageing 104
  concepts and definitions 104
  dementia 87, 94–97, 106–107

identifying and meeting
  health needs 104
Mental State
  Examination 108–109
promoting social
  inclusion 105
reducing health
  inequalities 104–105
role for learning disability
  nurses 104–105
oral hygiene 86, 88
oral medications 119
orthotics 101

pain 92–93, 107
palliative care 94–95
paracetamol 92, 119
parents with a learning
  disability 142–143
partnerships 116
Patau syndrome 14–15
patience 122
peer advocacy 148–149
perception assessment 109
personality disorder (PD) 68–69
person-centred care 51, 93, 122
person-centred planning
  family 134–135, 145
  implementation 135
  inclusion 134–135, 145
  role of learning disability
    nurse 135
  tools 135
pervasive developmental
  disorders (PDD) 56–57
phenylketonuria (PKU) 17, 23
physical abuse 36–37
physical examination 22
placements 7
play
  imaginary play 31
  learning through 30–31
  symbolic play 28–29
polypharmacy 115
post-traumatic stress disorder
  (PTSD) 151
postural care 100–101
Prader–Willi syndrome 14–15
pre-conception screening 22
pregnancy 142–143
pre-implantation testing 23
prescribing
  medications 116–117
primary healthcare
  facilitator 124–125
prison nurse 130–131
Prison Reform Trust 131
professional advocacy 148–149
professional values 4–5
Psychiatric Assessment
  Schedules for Adults with
  Developmental Disabilities
  (PAS-ADD) 51, 109

psychological distress 44–45
puberty 40–41
Public Sector Equality Duty 79
purist form of nursing 3

racism 42, 141
reasonable adjustments
  79, 137
receptive language 29, 52–53
recognition of child abuse 37
recognition of pain 92–93
religion 154
reminiscent work 107
residential options 138–139
respiratory illness 88–89
Rett syndrome 17
rights 122
Royal College of Nursing
  (RCN) 7, 99
Rubella 13, 26–27

safeguarding children 36–37
safety planning 101
scabies 26–27
schizophrenia 87, 89
school screening 22
screening 22–23, 34–35
seating for postural care 101
self-advocacy 148–149
sensorineural hearing loss 55
sensory impairment 54–55,
  87–89
serotonin and noradrenalin
  reuptake inhibitors
  (SNRIs) 112–113
serotonin reuptake inhibitors
  (SSRIs) 112–113
service development 123
service users 7, 146–147
sex and sexual health 98–99,
  152–153
sex education 152–153
sexism 42
sex-linked inheritance 23
sexual abuse 36–37, 153
Sexual Offences Act (2003)
  40, 98
shared consultation 116
sheltered workshops 136
sickle cell disease 23
signing 53
six Cs 6
Six Lives report (2009) 51
sizeism 42
sleep systems 101
Smith–Magenis
  syndrome 16–17
social care inequalities 141
social communication 29, 31,
  52–53
social inclusion *see* inclusion
social media 155–156
social networks 99

Special Educational Needs
  (SEN) 32–33
speech assessment 109
spirituality 154
standing frames 101
status epilepticus 59, 61
*Strengthening the Commitment
  Learning Disability Nursing*
  (CNO report) 3, 7
student nurses 7
SUDEP 58–59
Supervised Community
  Treatment (SCT) 81
supported living 139
support roles 2–3
swallowing problems 87
symbolic play 28–29

tablets 119
Tay–Sachs syndrome 17
teaching roles 123
team working skills 2, 4–5
thought assessment 109
thyroid disease 87
traffic light approach 92–93
training 40
transitions 46–47
tricyclic antidepressants
  (TCAs) 112–113
typical antipsychotics 112–113

understanding 28–29

Valuing Employment
  (2009) 137
Valuing People (2001) 47, 59
Valuing People Now (2009) 59,
  143
Varicella zoster 13, 26–27
verbal abilities 10
village communities 139
visual impairments 54–55,
  87–89
visual tools 53
voluntary work 134, 136
vulnerable adults 73–83
  Equality Act 78–79
  ethics, rights and
    responsibilities 82–83
  human rights 76–77, 83
  Mental Capacity Act 74–75
  Mental Health Act 80–81
  role of learning disability
    nurse 75, 77

Williams's syndrome 17
Winterbourne View Hospital
  report (2012) 51
work experience 136
work preparation schemes 136

young people with learning
  disability (YPwLD) 41